A LICENSE TO HEAL

Random Memories of an ER Doctor

STEVEN BENTLEY, M.D.

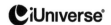

A LICENSE TO HEAL
RANDOM MEMORIES OF AN ER DOCTOR

iUniverse books may be ordered through booksellers or by contacting:

iUniverse LLC
1663 Liberty Drive
Bloomington, IN 47403
www.iuniverse.com
1-800-Authors (1-800-288-4677)

ISBN: 978-1-4917-3007-2 (sc)
ISBN: 978-1-4917-3008-9 (e)

Library of Congress Control Number: 2014906011

Printed in the United States of America.

iUniverse rev. date: 04/03/2014

For

My Brother: Michael – He taught me so much, and died too soon.

My Sister: Cheryl – For all the support, through all the years.

My Wife: Denise – The one who loved me, when no-one else could or would. She has provided me with encouragement, motivation, and the much needed computer skills, which enabled me to complete this project.

Contents

Introduction

My name is Steven Bentley. I am an American Board of Emergency Medicine board-certified ED doctor. These are some of the stories from my career over thirty-three years as an ER physician in North Carolina. It all started in the late 1970's, when I was in my early twenties.

In 1974, just a few years after the United States landed on the moon, while Watergate was causing a presidency to end and the late-night comedy "Saturday Night Live" was about to begin, I embarked on a career in medicine.

I am often asked why I chose medicine and the answer is fairly simple. I wanted to escape the poverty that I had known as a child. In addition, as a child, I had the opportunity to interact with many physicians, and came to know them as the *good guys*. I knew them as the people in the white coats, who made people feel better. I had the chance to interact with doctors because I have a birth defect known as "Kartagener's Syndrome". This syndrome is characterized by *situs inversus totalis* (all the internal organs of my body are reversed), *chronic bronchitis* (lung infections) and *chronic sinusitis* (sinus infections). I thought that if I had to work— and I did— then I might as well do something that was financially and intellectually rewarding, and medicine was all of that. Medical School was very difficult, and the field of medicine was not at all what I had expected it to be like. College had gone very well, and I even managed to win a few academic awards. Money was always hard to obtain. I assisted classes, worked for my father in his drug store, and labored at various other jobs, in order to pay the bills and school expenses. I had just gotten out of an orphanage and gone to live with my father. He had made it very clear that he was not going to help me financially, but this is too much about me and gets away from the stories that I became a part of in the emergency department.

As the years in medical practice rolled by, and the patient encounters accumulated, it became obvious that an emergency doctor has a rare observational vantage point from which to gain a perspective of the human experience. An ER doctor never knows what the next patient coming into the emergency room will have. I became aware of how privileged I was, and how interesting it might be to share these stories with others. These tales are all true, allowing for my memory. The names have been changed as required per discretion. I have chosen to present them in a linear fashion, beginning with my experiences in Medical School and proceeding through my career in the Emergency Department. I have deliberately neglected to relate personal experiences, because I wanted this book to be about the ER, and all the people that I had the privilege to meet.

One story, about a patients' near-death experience, seemed particularly important to share. This experience made an enormous impression on me. I am a scientific person. I am spiritual, but not at all religious. The experience of this patient will mean different things to different people, but I was there, and I know what I felt.

There were other stories, such as the young wife who lost her husband, and experienced a great deal of difficulty in accepting the loss or the young man who survived his auto accident, only to become suicidal. Learn of many other patients who were shot or stabbed, and how they coped. There were motor vehicle accidents that resulted in death or paralysis, as well as curious stories of "moonshine" and sometimes-unsettling personal revelations.

Travel with me, through medical school and medical training. Then, learn of the fascinating and very real world of emergency medicine, from the perspective of a working emergency physician. I do not have a degree from Harvard or Yale. I have a degree from a state school, the Medical College of Georgia, and I worked in the ER for thirty-three years. These are some of my stories.

CHAPTER 1

Opening Thoughts on Emergency Medical Practice

I WAS AT THE END OF my career, but I still had a few hard cases to attempt to solve as an emergency physician. This would be one of them. The hospital's emergency radio crackled and I heard the ambulance siren in the background. It was a sound that, as always, brought an uneasy suspense—because this call might require some rapid, large, life-saving interventions, or it may be nothing serious. The ambulance call came over the radio. The paramedics were bringing in a mid-thirty's male who had been shot in the left chest by the police during a store robbery.

Now, as the saying goes, it was -"*game on*". My mind made an intense shift into automatic-response mode to deal with the oncoming situation. As reported by the paramedics, the vital signs suggested early hypovolemic shock. His blood pressure was low and the pulse rate elevated, but he was still breathing on his own. They were administering normal saline fluid intravenously and were assisting his respirations with an Ambu bag.

Upon the patient's arrival, things moved quickly. A rapid exam confirmed the initial assessment. His blood pressure was 90/30, pulse 120. He was breathing on his own. There was an entrance bullet wound in the left upper chest, but no exit wound on the back was found. The wound was bleeding profusely.

This was a small community emergency department, so the trauma team consisted of me and the ER nurses— no other doctors. This has usually been the case in my career. We worked fast to stabilize the patient while quickly performing a secondary survey for any additional injuries. There were none.

Another IV was placed, and he was prepped for rapid sequence intubation. He was given versed and succinylcholine for paralysis and sedation. He was successfully intubated. When I listened with a stethoscope, the breath sounds were diminished in the left chest as I had expected. I inserted a large bore chest tube into the left chest— a tube thoracotomy. The chest tube was placed to drain any blood that might be present and to allow any potentially collapsed lung to expand.

Immediately, a large amount of blood gushed out onto the floor. Some towels were scattered around on the floor to keep from slipping in the blood. The chest tube was connected to a Pleur-evac. This is a plastic container for the collection of blood and/or air. I ordered a chest X-ray for tube position confirmation, and to locate the missing bullet.

After his x-ray had been taken and I was awaiting the results, I inserted a central line IV in the femoral vein of his right leg and began transfusing type specific blood from the lab. The patient had also been placed on a ventilator and was receiving 100% oxygen. The x-ray returned and demonstrated good tube position, with some blood remaining in the left chest. The bullet was seen in the left chest a little above the heart. Good lung expansion was noted. By this time the nurses had placed a Foley catheter in his bladder for urine drainage.

Next, we performed a reassessment. It showed some improvement in his vital signs and the blood oxygen, as measured by the pulse-oximeter, looked good. I began to breathe a little easier. I looked at the chest x-ray again for any pathology that I might have missed.

At about this time, the patient's BP began to fall. The IV fluid infusion was increased and more blood was transfused. He was too unstable to operate on and I was almost out of options. I ruled out a tension pneumothorax, a collapsed lung that impairs blood flow, and considered any further actions. I had none. He flat-lined and CPR was begun. Shortly thereafter, I pronounced him dead. This ended another patient encounter in the ER.

This episode caused me a lot of mental anguish. It probably should not have. The police were trying to kill him when they shot him, and he was robbing a store. I suspect that robbery is an inherently risky business. Maybe it was all the blood. There was a lot of blood. Perhaps I had seen too much death. It occurred to me that perhaps I was suffering from burn-out, even though personally, I am not even sure there is such a malady. In my despondency that day, I even pondered—after my decades of working in ER medicine— whether I was supposed to be an ER doctor. Burn-out was a possibility. I had all the classic symptoms. Another fact that I considered was that I had missed all the signs and symptoms of severe depression with suicidal ideation in my brother before his suicide. I was devastated. What if I was missing my own diagnosis?

Allow me a moment to explain a little bit about the rapidly evolving world of Emergency Medicine. In the old days (before the 1980's) there were no standards for the practice of Emergency Medicine. Anyone with an MD could work the emergency department and many doctors did. In those days it was very common for a doctor-in-training to "moonlight" in an emergency department somewhere to supplement his or her income. Unfortunately for the public, these physicians did not necessarily have any expertise in the area of medicine that a particular patient might need. For example, a patient may be having a heart attack and the "emergency physician" on that shift may be an Urologist, or a Dermatologist, or an Endocrinologist. There were no standards. The medical community recognized the need for a specialty in Emergency Medicine, and through the hard efforts of a few devoted individuals, it became a reality. Today, there are still some non-board certified physicians working in the field across the country, but they are becoming less common.

There is much controversy about whether board certified emergency physicians are any better than those physicians who are not board certified, but who have spent many years working in ER's. Even the terms *emergency room* and *emergency department* have generated heated debate, because some believe that the terms perpetuate negative stereotypes. The public widely knows the term emergency room, and

I am old now, so for the most part I will use that term. I had the good fortune to practice during these extremely interesting and changing times. The Chinese have an old saying *"may you live in interesting times"*, and I certainly have.

These are volatile times in the ER and medicine in general. Electronic Medical Records are coming and already in place in many hospitals. They may not work well in the ER setting, where the intensity of human need is too great and the pace too fast. They may become another documentation nightmare for emergency physicians. The idea is solid, and scribes may help (people who specialize in documenting on the charts, thus freeing the doctor to focus on the patients and not the chart).

I developed an interest in Emergency Medicine early in my medical training. I noticed that many of the doctors who came to give us lectures often started their discussion by saying "I was working in the ER when a patient came in" and then continue with whatever disease process they were trying to teach. I began to realize that if a person worked in the ER long enough, they would end up seeing most of the pathology that afflicts humans. I learned that this was true after a lifetime in the emergency department.

Everyone who walks or rolls into an emergency department wants something; the skilled ER physician can quickly assess what that is. The apparent patient may be there for work-related issues, litigation-related issues, chronic complaints, and many drug seekers. Hidden amongst this sea of patients are the truly ill and the truly dying. The trick is to decide which is which. Time is very short and there are so many patients. They all deserve to be seen, some sooner than others, but there is only one of you and many of them. It is my opinion that one of the most useful skills that an emergency physician can possess is the ability to rapidly assess a situation, and determine how critical each patient is.

It is fascinating, although disturbing, to hear the many deceptions and lies that people concoct in order to acquire narcotics. The task of ascertaining the truth is even more difficult when you discover that drug-seekers have hijacked legitimate medical problems in order to make the story more convincing. Chronic back pain, migraines, renal stones and multiple sclerosis are a few of the many conditions that drug-seekers try to simulate. The red flag is that these patients are always allergic to every pain killer, except the one drug that they are trying to obtain. I saw one man who was so desperate for opiates that he would even have abdominal surgery to obtain IV Morphine.

It is infuriating to witness the limited medical resources being hijacked by ER abusers. For example, suppose there are only three ambulances in the county, but two of them are tied up transporting chronic problems or young people with headaches and they could have safely made it to the ER on their own. If your family member has a heart attack or is in a car wreck there might be no one left to provide immediate assistance. The paramedics often tell me that there were multiple cars in the driveway, but the patients say they did not want to use their own gasoline. They often add that they did not try any aspirin or Tylenol for the headache, but just came to the ER for a "shot". We were never taught about this in medical school.

There is another reason that ER was so appealing. The practice of emergency medicine involves people in acute situations by definition. It may be anything from gunshot wounds, chainsaw injuries, car crashes, diabetic coma, heart attack or kidney failure. What is truly humbling and impressive is the scope of human illness— both triumphant and tragic— that an emergency medicine physician is allowed to help with.

Hopefully, the ER physician can intervene, and steer the situation in a positive direction. Occasionally, one encounters a patient *in extremis*— on the verge of dying from whatever cause. It is extremely gratifying if you are then able to draw on your knowledge and skill and improve the situation—sometimes averting death. It is such a fantastic feeling of elation to watch them as they realize that they are better and all their family members gather close to see for themselves. I am sure that this feeling of elation occurs in many other fields of endeavor, but I found it in the emergency room. Several times I have seen patients who thought they were going to die, revive and find life again. It really feels wonderful.

On several occasions I have thwarted the death of patients who thought they were going to die—sometimes I literally resuscitated them. It is truly a spectacular feeling. Acute pulmonary edema (fluid on the lungs) is just such a diagnosis. The patient may present gasping for breath, sweat pouring off of them, and a feeling of impending death. In 30-45 minutes, the physician can dramatically improve the situation and make the patient feel so much better.

Just like most people, I have experienced many different personal issues through the years, such as death in the family, divorce, and failed relationships. I have tried my best not to let them distract me from providing the best possible care for my patients. I have often heard about Bill Clinton's ability to "compartmentalize" his life—focusing on one thing at a time without distraction. I think most people are able to do this to some extent. I have found this ability invaluable in my life. I have attempted, in my career, to "check my personal baggage" at the ER door at the start of a shift.

While I focused on serving my patients, expanding my knowledge and experience, and honing my physician skills, the business structures of medical practice were changing around me. I became extremely tired of the constant emphasis on profit demonstrated by the large health-care corporations that now control emergency departments. I received many derogatory e-mails from the corporate office stating that I had not generated enough income for them during the past quarter, and suggesting that perhaps I should order more unnecessary test, or admit more patients unnecessarily, since that was where the money was in medicine. I asked if I had missed any diagnoses, and they replied no, but I had not made them enough money. I responded that I had not gone into medicine in order to make profits for them. I was even told once that I no longer see patients, but that I see customers. I realized that the practice of medicine had changed radically and that I had not changed with it. So I quit.

I have often heard that "the USA has the best healthcare system" in the world. I suspect that Switzerland, Sweden, Denmark, Germany, Brazil and many other nations would disagree with this assertion. I can say that the healthcare system is trying very hard to be the best, but what good is it to be the best if nobody can afford it? I have heard comments about all the physicians leaving the field. The people that are opposed to the Affordable Care Act generally blame President Obama for this.

In my experience, there may be some physicians who are leaving because of financial limitations. But I also have seen that many are disappointed with the changes in medical practice that require them to see more patients in less time, and not to spend too much time with any one patient because that interferes with the profit. They also frequently cite the increase in litigation as a factor in their decision to quit. It makes a hard job even harder when the physician views each patient encounter as a potential litigation case and not just a sick human being.

The practice of emergency medicine is different from office practice in many ways. In the ER, there are no scheduled patients. It would be nice if they would spread out the visits over the day, but they tend to come in clusters. The shifts are for twelve straight hours (When I started, the shifts were 24 hours long). In my case, I usually have been the sole doctor available to cover all walk-ins as well as ambulance arrivals. There are no breaks, just twelve straight hours of emergency medicine. Some patients are dying faster than others, and it is your job to decide which is which. Many cases involve a large quantity of unknowns.

Compared to a doctor's general practice, emergency medicine raises the stakes in two ways: the acuteness or severity of the conditions is higher, and so is the trauma or misery. The acuity is high and so are the malpractice rates. On the other hand, when you are off, you are completely off, unlike many of the primary care givers I have known. Then I could read, bike, jog or catch up on life without being on-call. In comparison, think of the frustration that a general surgeon must feel when he or she is called by the ER. Often, they spend a great deal of time trying to repair someone who has been injured, but will never pay them. Then, they have to go operate on the scheduled patients who have often waited weeks for their surgery. General surgeons must be so exhausted.

I have learned that in the practice of Emergency Medicine, it is necessary to learn how to function in the "automatic mode". It is necessary because it is too easy to be swept away in the drama, gore and excitement of the moment and forget some very important step in patient management. One of the first things that an ER doctor needs to learn is that *"it is not your blood"*. It is extremely important to be able to focus on the patient and not become distracted by all the commotion. If the doctor becomes distracted or unfocused, then the patient will lose. As an example, I remember an incident where the paramedics brought in a victim from a car wreck. The patient was covered with a sheet and there was blood all over. As they moved the patient from the stretcher to the bed, his legs fell off onto the floor. I was shocked. What could I possibly do for this poor man? I was horrified and it showed on my face. The patient saw my expression and began laughing. "They are just prosthetic legs, doc. Don't get upset" he chuckled. Stay focused. This is where all the training and all the Emergency Education courses come into play. They all stress repetition and rigorous attention to protocol. If it seems repetitious, that's because it is.

Another huge benefit to emergency medicine is that we, the physicians, are paid by a third party. This means that we don't have to worry about our patient's ability to pay for our time. We can order lab tests and x-rays as we feel they are indicated and useful. We can practice as much, or as little, medicine as we feel is necessary for that particular patient. I enjoyed this aspect of EM enormously. Most primary care physicians do not have this luxury.

I know the argument about "*the highly paid*" doctors. Physicians indeed are well compensated for their time. I personally never made more than $200,000.00 in a year, but I always felt very well-off. I suppose that it depends on your definition of *rich*. I once heard someone say that "being rich" meant that he did not have to worry when the car would break down. I agree with that concept. After all, while one might attain a fine home and expensive food, a person can only be so dry and so well-fed. There are some other jobs that pay more than a physician's does. No doctor that I know has ever made the millions that are paid to the CEO's of Fortune 500 companies or professional athletes. Moreover, the CEO's don't take call, work the holidays, and are not exposed to the high incidence of medical litigation. While we are on the subject, no Nobel Prize winners and very few scientists make the large money either. I suppose that is the *free market* at work.

Every story has a beginning, and so does this one. The story opens in the Medical College of Georgia, my medical school.

CHAPTER 2

Medical School

ALLOW ME A MOMENT TO EXPLAIN how Medical School was structured when I went to school. The first two years of school are spent in the classroom, with such topics as general anatomy, cell and molecular biology, histology, pathology and many more. During the final 2 years, the student traveled to the wards, where they began to see real patients and learn how to apply all of that knowledge. If it all goes well, now the student graduates and becomes an MD.

Then, a marathon of learning begins with the internship. The student may then select a field of pursuit and start their residency in their field. It may be general medicine, general surgery or general pediatrics. If they choose they can continue with one of the subspecialties such as pulmonary medicine, gastroenterology, cardiology or perhaps one of the surgical subspecialties such as orthopedic surgery, thoracic surgery, ENT surgery, and many others. During the internship and residency years, the student becomes part of a team.

A team usually consists of an attending physician, a resident, 2 interns and 4 medical students. The attending is usually an accomplished physician, in their specialty, and has joined the faculty of the Medical School. The responsibility, and therefore the liability, is arranged in the following manner: the attending is responsible for all medical decisions made on the patients on his service. Next in line is the resident. They are also responsible for all decisions and actions on the patients on their service and answers directly to the attending. Then, there are the interns. They divide the patients equally between them and assume all the day to day care and decisions on each patient. They answer to the resident. Finally, there are the medical students. They have no real responsibility or liability, since they are students, not doctors. However, they do an enormous amount of work. It is often referred to as "scut" work, which simply means all the "leg" work and basic patient care that others do not have time to do such as chasing down lab work, starting intra-venous lines, getting x-rays, feeding patients, following up on consults and much more. This is the way it was organized when I went to school 35 years ago, obviously it may have changed.

At first, I thought I had made a huge mistake in pursuing medicine because of the following stories. In my earlier education, I really loved the sciences and in particular biology. The message, over the medical school lecture hall door, quoted Dante's Inferno – *"Abandon hope, all ye who enter here"*. A bit dramatic, but I got the message.

My study partner (he will return later in the story) introduced himself, and then proceeded to tell me that his goals were to "screw a different girl each night" and "drive a Ferrari" by the time he graduated. The only thing that came to my mind, was that I thought it was a good thing to have goals.

A significant negative experience occurred when one of the scheduled lectures was on female anatomy. The large medical class, consisting mostly of young males, began to laugh, and hoot. They made loud, obnoxious commentary to the professor, who was obviously very shy and having quite enough trouble with the subject as it was. He was an Amish man. I am not a prude, but he was having a hard enough time as it was and I felt sorry for him. They acted like hormonally stimulated high school kids. I guess I expected more maturity. I was mistaken.

I am not sure who at medical school chooses what students must study and learn, but in looking back it seems very arbitrary and not in line with basic, daily practice at all. By the time I graduated, I was sure that glycogen-storage (enzyme diseases affecting the liver) diseases were rampant. Yet, after thirty-three years of practice I have never seen a case. I knew almost nothing about everyday coughs, colds, or infant feedings and bowel movements, but I did learn. On the job training as it were.

Medical school was not so bad after all. We had note-taking service and I had someone to get all the hand-outs for me, so I cut a lot of classes and showed up for the tests. I found the lectures to be very tedious and I discovered that attending class wasn't really necessary, so I would go to the local lake and swim. I made very good grades, so I was satisfied. I thought of writing a book titled *How to Go to Medical School in Your Spare Time*. One of my classmates left a note in my mailbox that read "please come back to class, we all miss you".

An x-ray of my chest was often used as a teaching tool for the medical students, because of my Kartagener's Syndrome. The CXR shows my heart shadow on the opposite side and all the students would approach the viewing screen and reverse the film, to show the instructor they were paying attention to detail. The instructor would promptly inform them that this x-ray portrayed a patient with Kartagener's Syndrome (me) and that the heart shadow was correct in this case. It always got a few laughs from the class.

After the first two years of classroom at medical school, we began to rotate through the primary care services such as General Medicine, General Surgery, Pediatrics, and a few subspecialties. The schools tend to rotate the students through the different specialties in order to provide a broader view of medical care.

My first rotation was Pediatrics. When we arrived on the wards at the hospital, after the first two years of books, I was terrified. I knew almost nothing about fevers, infant formulas, normal weights. This was a referral center. A referral center is a hospital that has staffing in all the specialties and subspecialties. The facility usually accepts patients from all across the state, who have exhausted all the local physicians' abilities to help that patient. All the children had strange, fatal diseases and they were so small.

On my first day, I watched a terrible pediatric code blue. The child was a year and a half old and ceased breathing and his heart stopped. The resident could not get the endo-tracheal tube in and lacerated the child's mouth trying to accomplish this task. In the meantime, we still used intra-cardiac epinephrine, so another resident stuck his heart, punctured his lung, and gave him massive subcutaneous emphysema (an air pocket under the skin) before everyone quit and the child was pronounced dead. I was frightened and nauseated by the frantic, violent young death. Things didn't look good for me.

There were many other heart-rending stories as well. One little boy had a very aggressive cancer and was going to die. He and I used to go outside to eat lunch, and so that he could be out of the hospital for a little while. He had to have a lot of blood drawn for tests, and I would hold his nose so they could get the blood. He liked that. I don't know why.

I quickly learned that some of the long-time nurses knew a lot of medicine. I learned a lot of solid medicine from the experienced, seasoned nurses that I have been fortunate enough to work with in my career. I was in the hospital now, which is how most medical schools arrange their scheduling. I was now in my early 20's. I met an older nurse on the ward named Lucy. She took me under her wing and taught me a lot of practical medicine. Once I had an actively seizing patient and I needed to give him some IV Magnesium. I was scrambling trying to convert milliequivalents to milligrams, when Lucy said "Just give him an amp". I was scared and asked if she were sure. "Yes, just give him an amp" she replied. It worked, and I was amazed.

Lucy taught me so many valuable things: How to dress a wound. The way to start an IV, and the proper way to irrigate Foley catheters. The way to put down NG tubes (a plastic tube inserted through the nose for feeding and suction). She also taught me to find out how they liked the food, whether they had eaten, and what they missed the most. These were the most practical things to know. I really appreciated Lucy.

Being on the wards was both frightening and fascinating. There was so much to learn and I always felt like I just did not know enough. I once ordered a single dose of Indocin (similar to Motrin) for pain. The patients kidneys started to fail and another student suggested that it was because of the Indocin. I was shocked. I thought, *One oral dose of medicine for pain and I killed his kidneys*! I read up on NSAID drugs (like Motrin) and found that they could indeed result in decreased glomerular filtration (blood flow to the kidneys) although usually at higher doses and not very often.

The patient eventually did just fine but now I was afraid to give anything. I did not know every possible side effect of every drug! No one did. It took a while to calm down. Meanwhile, the patients kept on coming, and the problems got bigger.

I had a patient named Charlie. He was my first patient to die. I took care of Charlie for several weeks. We got to know each other and became friends. He had a type of leukemia and had already been through all the known treatments. He had a wonderful family. His death was prolonged, painful and agonizing. Toward the end, the resident and intern pretty much gave up on him, but I—the student— wanted him to make it.

One night he began bleeding from all his orifices. His urine, rectum, nose and some vomit contained blood. He was hurting so much and kept asking for more morphine. I just kept giving it to him. I tried to help, but there was nothing left to do. He died.

I attended his autopsy. My school encouraged attendance at autopsies. It was the last one I ever went to. There was my friend, cut open on a table with his chest lying on his face. He was all cut up. No more laughing and joking. I am glad someone does these things, but it is best not to know the individual. I already knew why he died and it pained me to see him that way. His family wrote me a very nice letter of thanks later. I still have that after all these years.

The wards were a lot of hard work and a jarring introduction to real human sickness. No more lectures and notes, just real people with real diseases. I was a 4th year student and feeling smug— a little knowledge can do that. I went into a female patient's room to perform the new patient interview and exam. She was a very large woman. She was lying on the bed and spilling over both sides. The head of the bed was partially raised so that we could talk.

I introduced myself and asked her why she had come to the hospital. She replied that she had lost her appetite. At this, we both began to laugh. I told her that I thought it was the best thing that had ever happened to her. Perhaps it was not the most professional comment, but she accepted it, and we just kept laughing. Now in her defense, there are indeed some unpleasant diagnoses that result in the person losing their appetite and gaining weight, but we both thought this was too funny.

I finished my interview and performed my comprehensive "student physical exam". The complete exam required a pelvic exam. The examination room was down the hall, so I helped her into a wheelchair to roll her down to exam room. The room was at the end of a long hallway that, unfortunately for me, had a slight uphill incline to it. I proceeded up the incline, but it was getting much more difficult to push her. She was so large that the sides of the wheelchair were pushed out against the wheels and acting like brakes. I was pushing and straining and breathing harder. I am sure it was very comical to witness. One of my fellow students passed me in the hall going the opposite direction. After he passed, and she could no longer see him, he doubled over in laughter with tears on his face. I was determined to finish the job. We finally arrived at the pelvic room.

I helped her get out of the chair and onto the examining table. These tables are uncomfortable under the best of circumstances, and this was less than ideal. I performed the exam, but I was too young and inexperienced to know that because she was so large, the exam would be futile. In retrospect, it was all a big waste of time and was extremely unpleasant and uncomfortable for her. Fortunately for her the work-up was negative and we never found an etiology for the loss of appetite.

Several weeks later, the scene had changed, and I was serving a different patient in another part of the hospital. I was in Labor and Delivery, and this patient was in active labor. She was screaming and rolling around in pain. In those days we used a drug called Scopolamine for pain control. It can induce a form of amnesia. She had been given Scopolamine, and was going wild with the contractions. She reached out and grabbed my inner thigh and began to grope for my groin, screaming "you *son-of-bitch*, you did this to me". I jumped back and yelled that "I didn't do it— don't hurt me". She calmed down and the rest of the delivery went well.

Another time, I had just finished delivering a baby, when the nurse said "I think there is another one". This was before routine ultrasound, and this patient had not received any prenatal care. I had never delivered twins. At first I thought the nurse was joking with me, but then I realized that she was serious.

I ran back, examined the patient, and thought, *damn, she is right, there is another baby*. Fortunately, the second delivery went well and everyone was happy. I was so scared again.

It seems like I spent so much time being afraid. I was always afraid that things would not turn out well, or that I did not know enough. The fear, for me, only began to dim with time and experience. It has always fascinated me how different people, in many different situations, cope with their pain in such distinctly different ways. Some are very quiet and withdrawn, while others scream like a Banshee.

Perhaps some doctor's deal with the job stress by driving too fast. Remember my study partner. He and I had been together on this OB rotation in Columbus, Georgia. We finished and headed back to Augusta. He had a very nice convertible sports car, and I was driving another old, used VW Beetle. I had driven many VW "bugs" because they were so inexpensive to buy and drive. He passed me on the highway, laughing and waving. My car would not go very fast. A few miles up the road, I passed him, pulled over on the side of the road. The Highway Patrol had caught him speeding and had him pulled over. I don't think I ever felt so good about a traffic ticket.

I got back from OB, and immediately began a Neurosurgery rotation. This was a big waste of time in my opinion. The neurosurgeons never even learned our names and never discussed the cases, or the reasoning behind the therapy that was chosen. We didn't have any smart, kind neurosurgeons, like CNN's Dr. Sanjay Gupta, on this service.

It is funny to watch rounds, because there is a distinct hierarchy to the walking pattern. There are all these white coats marching down the hall together. At the head is the attending, then the residents, then the interns, and at last the students. It must be very difficult to be a patient at a teaching hospital and have a large group of strange doctors come to your room each day, stand at the end of the bed, and discuss your case.

The neurosurgeons in charge treated us as unwanted baggage and all we did on the rotation was run down lab work and x-rays, often referred to as "scut-work". We were making rounds one morning, when they entered a patient's room. The patient was a midforties woman who had a life, a husband and three kids. She was informed that her tests had come back and they suggested that she had a glioblastoma—a type of very aggressive brain cancer. This particular diagnosis has a very bad prognosis or outcome. They informed her that they would like to put her on the surgery schedule for the next day. She hesitated and began to cry. They became impatient and again insisted that she needed to sign consent for the operation the next day.

She was having a great deal of difficulty trying to process all the information and was terribly confused. All she could do was cry. She was very afraid and very alone. She had just been given a death sentence and not given any time to talk with her husband. She was extremely sad and so very scared. She cried that she would never get to see her children grow up. I told the neurosurgery team that I would stay behind, get the form signed, and catch up with them. They agreed and left.

I held her and tried to explain what her diagnosis was and what it meant. She had never even heard of a glioblastoma. I talked with her for a long time and told her that there was no hurry on the operation and that she should certainly talk with her husband first. I felt so sorry for her. I caught up with the team and told them that she wanted to hold off and discuss things with her husband. They cursed because the surgery was delayed and went on with rounds. She agreed to have the surgery a few days later. The lady died a few months later.

Another day, and another rotation. This time I was on psychiatry. I never cared for psychiatry. Once you made a diagnosis, all you could really do is talk to the patient and try to get them to modify their behavior. I guess I did not like the lack of control over the situation. You did not have the option of giving them a particular form of therapy and making them better. You simply had to point out the problem and hope they could modify their behavior in order to make life better. This type of patient accounted for most of psychiatry patients. Then, there were the severely ill patients with psychoses, like schizophrenia and true manic-depression. There were some medications that would help, but by and large, it is still an area of medicine that is very mysterious and unknown.

I had one patient, on my psychiatry rotation, who was a fourteen year old girl from Charleston, S.C. Her parents were married and her father was a dentist. She was very depressed and had already tried to commit suicide several times. She was very intelligent and easy to talk with. We developed a close relationship during our sessions. I remember trying to discuss the case with my resident, but he was so strung out on drugs that any meaningful discussion was impossible.

I finally had a chance to meet the young girl's parents one day. No wonder she had a problem. They argued from the first moment I met them. They pushed each other and argued over who was going to speak to the doctor first. I just watched and then tried to discuss the case with them and go over possible solutions. They continued to argue among themselves.

At last, the father turned to me and offered to give the girl to me for the summer. I did not know what to say. As I saw it, I was a young, hormonal male who barely knew the girl, much less the parents. This proffered solution, such as it was, had no chance of benefiting the young girl. I said no, of course. My resident and attending were of no use in this situation. I continued to talk with the young girl.

I rotated off psychiatry, but continued to check on her case. She succeeded in committing suicide a few months later. I was truly sorry for her.

Sometimes, odd behavior could be found among the physician population. While I was on this rotation, we had weekly conferences with all the leading physicians, of this department, to discuss therapeutic options for our patients. One time, as we were all gathered in the large conference room around a huge wooden table the chief physician excused himself to go to the restroom. The restroom was a small room right off the conference room. He went in, left the door wide open, and began to urinate. This conference consisted of a mixed gender group, and he was in full view of all the physicians at the table. It was a bit awkward. This was a referral-center hospital. It seemed extremely odd to me.

Prior to completing my training, I rotated onto general medicine. The patients were very sick and there was a variety of pathology to learn from. One afternoon, all the house-staff, other than me and a few other students, had gone to another hospital for the regularly scheduled Morbidity and Mortality conference. While all the real doctors were gone, a patient came in with severe upper gastrointestinal bleeding. He was vomiting large amounts of blood.

We began doing all the interventions that we had learned. We placed two large IV's with Ringer's lactate, placed a Foley catheter, and drew blood for routine tests as well as type and cross-matched blood. We began the blood transfusions and performed gastric lavage (washing out the stomach) with ice water to slow the bleeding and clear the stomach. We don't do this anymore because no studies have demonstrated that it is beneficial. It seemed to be a pretty savage treatment even then. The patient was improving and we felt pretty good about things. Then my resident returned from his conference. His only response was to quip "two times zero is still zero". This implied that since we were just students, nothing had really been done for this patient. This made me so incensed that I exploded and hit him in the face. I did not hit him hard. I just blacked his eye, and bloodied his nose. He had been abusing us for weeks. I know that what I had done was not right, but I was really angry. Nothing was ever said about the incident and I just dropped the issue. We were very scared, as students, and had done all this work. The patient had gotten better, heck-we might have even saved his life, and that was all that the resident had to say to us. No— "thanks, good job", just ridicule. I refused to ever work with that resident again.

I was on general medicine, at the VA hospital. I was learning, but still had a long, long way to go. I was living in a local apartment. My life consisted of sleeping, eating and working shifts.

One of my patients was a man named Juddie. He was a tall, imposing man even though he was in his ninety's. Juddie had a bad habit of stealing food from the other patients. Many of the patients were bed-ridden and could not get up. This was the old VA hospital and the rooms, back in those days, had four beds in them. After the food was served, he would wait until the staff was absent. Then he would wander over to one of the bed-ridden patient's tray table and roll it away. They would protest, but they could not do anything. He would just laugh and take the tray back to his table to eat. I finally caught him, but I could not make him stop. He would just laugh at me.

One of my classmates was a smart, professional woman, but she was very religious as well as naïve. One day she had an exam to perform on one of the male patients. She finished her history and physical, and came to the final part of the physical - the genital exam. In an extremely professional and dignified manner, she asked him to expose his genitals for the exam. He looked at her and said "that is all you women want to do is take it out and play with it". I burst into laughter. She blushed, began to cry, and then ran out of the room. After we calmed her down, she was able to return and finish the exam. You have to learn.

A different time, one of my male patients was getting hemo-dialysis (blood-purification to treat failing kidneys).

This procedure was unpleasant for the patients, and extremely boring. They usually had the procedure three times per week. This day, the dialysis nurse ran down the hall to tell me that my patient was masturbating. I just laughed and told her if it bothered her, then just throw a blanket over him. I was learning.

Another day, and another rotation. The patient was an elderly man who was having trouble swallowing. His work-up revealed an esophageal carcinoma - cancer of the esophagus. This particular diagnosis had a terrible prognosis and no good treatment options. He taught me a lot about terminal patients. Before the diagnosis, he had been a drinker and a womanizer. Now he had "seen the light" and decided to get religion—give up drinking, smoking and women. This was how he had lived for the last 40 or 50 years. If he was going to improve his life, perhaps he should have done it a few years earlier. While I knew that this was the "bargaining" phase of dying, it was difficult to watch.

It was his decision to make, but I did not want to see him spend his last few months on this earth sick and in pain from the chemotherapy and radiation therapy. The therapy would give him another month or two at best, but there would be no quality of life. Many dying people will grasp at any chance at all, no matter what the consequences. As I said, it was his choice to make.

I got so angry with the Oncologists that I knew. They were very driven people and would often present the treatment options in such a way as to downplay the negative side effects, such as sickness, pain, and hair loss, while they played up the possible gains of extended life. The patients had never seen someone spend six of their remaining eight weeks vomiting, retching, and feeling bad all the time. They often grabbed at the promise of "more life", but what a cost!

As I have learned, many people decide that they do not wish to have any extreme interventions at the end, such as intubation and ventilation. The problem is that they make these decisions when they are still well, sitting around the kitchen table. It seems so noble, but when their time, comes the ambulance races down the highway with sirens screaming, heading for the ER. They can't breathe, their eyes are staring ahead with wild anxiety and the sweat is rolling off of them. Death is staring them in the face. Then, they often change their minds. It is only human nature. It can be a real dilemma when the accompanying family tells you not to do anything because that is what the patient had told them. Now, however, he or she has changed their mind and they are "of sound mind". The general principle is that a patient controls their own medical choices and can change their mind.

I have learned a great deal from the terminally ill patients that I have had the honor of knowing. I now have a "living will", and have expressed my strong desire not to have any heroic efforts applied to me to prolong life, and no ventilators please.

Speaking of radiation therapy— that is a great occupation. I used to watch the Radiation Oncologists come to work late, driving their Porsches. They would break early for lunch, stay late, roll back in, then leave early. They did not work weekends, holidays, or take call. Instead, the radiation technicians did most of the hard work with the patients. If I sound jealous, it is because I was jealous.

The private practice of dermatology is another low-key specialty. At least dermatology is somewhat interesting at a tertiary medical center where a doctor might see leprosy and other exotic diseases. In private practice, it is mostly acne, psoriasis and the occasional melanoma.

Also, it was often the best in the class who became these specialists. This angered me. We needed those very smart people in the ER, on the front lines, but that is just my opinion. After all, the ER was frantic, hard and required a lot of sacrifice. Ultimately, who can say whether these specialists made the right choice? Primary practice and surgery were even worse.

I went to Grady Hospital in Atlanta, Georgia to do my Emergency Dept. rotation. This is where I fell in love with emergency medicine. The ED was so large that it was divided into departments. There was general medicine, surgery, gynecology and obstetrics, and finally pediatrics.

I was assigned to the surgical department. I walked into the department and approached the resident to introduce myself and check-in. My white "doctor" coat had pockets that were full of books on "How to be a Doctor". The resident had his back to me, and was furiously writing on an ER exam sheet. A patient was behind him with his hand in a Styrofoam cup. The fingers were severed and the hand was bleeding profusely. I was shocked. The patient kept trying to get the resident's attention, but to no avail. The resident just spoke without even turning around. "Do you have a blue card? We can't see you without a blue card". I was appalled. It seemed so cold.

Another patient was in the corner of the ER, handcuffed to a chair. A police officer was with him, but currently was occupied, as he tried to hit on one of the nurses. The handcuffed patient began to have a seizure, but no one even paid attention. After the seizure, he regained consciousness and began to try and escape, but he could not get the chair through the door. I made the officer aware of his prisoner's escape attempt and the officer quickly intervened.

Meanwhile, the patient with the bloody hand had been escorted back to a room. More patients continued to pour into the ED. I loved it. The chaos was exciting, and there was so much action. It was so stimulating, exhilarating and incredibly interesting. The residents were not really callous, they had just seen so much stuff. In two months, I was acting much the same way.

In the winter a lot of "homeless" people would check-in and try to get admitted, to get a hot meal and get out of the cold. You couldn't blame them, but the hospital had a much different purpose. As Bob Dylan said "*if you ain't got nothing, you got nothing to lose*". One determined patient tried to get admitted for vomiting blood. His work-up was completely negative and his admission was refused. He then went outside, swallowed some razor blades and came back. Alright, the ER said, this time he could be admitted. A bit extreme, but it worked.

The Emergency Department and its surrounding area was a focal point of activity—some humorous, some tragic. All ambulances coming to the ER drove under an overpass next to the ED's bay. On the overpass sat a group of local "street people". As the ambulances pulled up to the ED, they would cheer the patients on with encouraging shouts. They became known as "Grady Rooters". In contrast, there a lady was raped in the Rape Crisis Center and one of the housestaff was shot on the sidewalk a few blocks from the hospital.

I really loved the excitement of the ER, but I did not spend absolutely all of my time there. One evening, I was relaxing in a jazz-bar up in Buckhead. A song came over the sound system that I did not recognize. I thought to myself "That was pretty good; I'll bet he does well". The song was "*Born to Run*" and, of course, the artist was Bruce Springsteen. Yeah, I think he did alright.

CHAPTER 3

Training—Internship and Residency

I FINALLY FINISHED MEDICAL SCHOOL IN 1978. I began my internship year. My God, I was terrified. One day you are not responsible for anything, because the intern is always responsible, and the very next day you are responsible for everything. It was truly overwhelming, and I really don't think anything can prepare you psychologically for the incredible feeling of responsibility. I had taken all the right courses and done all the right things, but now I was an *intern*, a real doctor. *Oh my God!* I thought. *What if I don't know enough? What if I kill somebody?*

Fear is an important emotion. Enough fear can motivate a doctor to learn more, try harder, and improve patient care. Too much fear can paralyze a physician, and make him ineffective. No fear can result in arrogance and patient mistakes with bad outcomes for the patient. I personally, had a lot of fear early in my career and then much less with the passage of time, as I accumulated knowledge and experience.

The fear is generated by many factors. Sometimes it is a fear of the unknown. There is so much information to know. Sometimes it is the one-upmanship that is so common in medical school — pretending to know more facts and gain favor with the attending. Often the fear is simply being afraid of causing pain in another human being. Many decisions that we, as physicians, are responsible for have the potential to cause enormous physical and psychological pain to our patients. I often speak of being afraid in these stories. This is what I am speaking about.

The fear was mixed with pride. We were all very proud to finally be doctors. We had arrived. We had made it. At first, a lot of us were filled with youthful optimism and enthusiasm for healing the sick masses of the world. After about 3 months, we were no longer optimistic, and all of the enthusiasm was gone. A heavy dose of *"Reality"* and the seemingly unending shifts had taken all that out of us. Now, when I looked around, I could see a lot of exhausted, sleep-deprived individuals whose lives had been reduced to simple survival. The shifts were 12 hours, 12 hours, then 36 hours on, for months on end. The unending stream of patients, with a variety of pathologies to learn about, was becoming unbearable. The starched white coats, with pockets full of "How to Be a Doctor" books, that had been so prevalent at the start, were now rumpled and stained. The books had been replaced by the ubiquitous and practical "Washington Manual of Medical Therapeutics" (a textbook that many physicians use).

I could not help but notice the similarities to a long march. At first, the participants are eager and hopeful, but after a few miles they change, and begin to discard various items, until at last they are down to the essentials. I noticed about 12 years ago that they finally began to limit the hours that a doctor-in training could work per week to 85. That is still a very respectable work load, but at least it is a step in the right direction. If I were a patient, I would want a rested, fresh doctor helping me or my family. Not the one who had already worked 30 or more hours.

The nurses were so funny. They knew that all of us were scared, and when they would address us they would say sarcastically "what would you like to do-Doctor?" I spent the next few months scrambling, trying to care for patients, not kill anyone, and quickly learn about their disease processes. An interesting dynamic in all of this is how each person deals with his or her pathologic process. As I discovered, a lot of being a doctor is simply trying to help the individual cope with their own personal process or tragedy. I spent a lot of time on the general medicine wards because I had discovered that the really sick patients were there, so it was an enormous opportunity for a lot of learning.

I was right. One particular patient stands out. He was a large male in his mid-sixties. He suffered a heart attack that caused him to rupture the *chordae tendonae* (a heart cord that holds one of the heart valves). This resulted in acute heart failure secondary to acute aortic regurgitation (back-flow of the blood in the heart when the valve won't close correctly). He was a very nice man who had a very bad disease with a horrible prognosis. Each day, I would go into his room and examine him and come to the same conclusion. His heart failure was getting worse, and without an operation to repair or replace the valve he was going to die. We would talk and I tried to explain to him what was happening to his body. He was so severe now that he had to remain in the sitting position all the time or he could not breathe due to the heart failure.

My Thoracic Surgeons agreed with the diagnosis and the fatal prognosis, but they were unwilling to try and help. They were afraid that he would die on the operating table and of course that would make their statistics look bad. They were right to be afraid. He was so severe that he had a good chance of dying on the table, but without the operation he was surely going to die. I was frantic. We started to joke among ourselves that we had the only "non-invasive surgeons" around. Every day when I examined him, he was a little worse and a little weaker. I wanted badly to help this man, but my options were very limited.

I called a hospital in Birmingham, Alabama and spoke with the Thoracic Surgeon there. After a few short minutes he said "sounds like your man needs an operation". I was ecstatic! Yes, I agreed but my surgeons would not help. He replied "if you can get him to me, we will do it". *Alright!* I spent the next several hours arranging all the logistics for the transfer and flight. I explained to the man what I was doing and why. He agreed.

I saw him a few weeks later, walking around at the Master's Golf Tournament. It was Augusta, Georgia after all. It was wonderful to see him alive, well and walking. We shook hands and laughed. Sometimes, it actually does work out well.

I feel compelled to tell you about a man named Solomon Darby. I have thought about this man many times over the last thirty-five years or so. It was truly a very profound experience for me. Mr. Darby was a patient of mine on the general medicine wards during my training. Solomon was an older, African American with a mouth full of gold teeth. He was a personable man. His smile would light up the room, but he did not smile much. He had been admitted with a large lung mass that was probably cancer, but we needed to find out which one it was so that a treatment regimen could be planned. I was extremely busy, and he was just one of many patients on the ward. Every morning we would round on him and ask how he was doing. He would always reply that he was doing well.

One day, after rounds, it came to my attention that Solomon could not move his legs. Indeed, as it turned out he was paralyzed from the waist down. I was incredulous. I asked him why he had not said something during rounds. He just replied that I had not asked him specifically about his legs.

As we move quickly to address this issue, it became obvious that the lung mass was probably cancer and it was now encroaching on his thoracic spinal cord, causing the paralysis. It is called "cord syndrome". I had not seen it before. He needed immediate radiation to the tumor in an attempt to shrink it and save the spinal cord. We accomplished this and he responded well, with resumption of motion and feeling in his legs. I was so glad, and began to pay him much more attention at rounds each day.

As I have already alluded to, Mr. Darby most likely had a lung cancer, but we were not sure of the type. I suspected he was dying. One day, during rounds, we entered his room. Solomon had is arms up in the air, stretched out in front of him, with the hands cocked back. He had his eyes open and it seemed that he was looking at something or someone far away. He was smiling that broad, bright smile of his. He did not seem to pay attention to our group as we approached but just kept staring off into the distance. In a pleasant tone, he spoke to people that I could not see.

I asked him how he was doing and he said just fine, he continued by saying "I don't need no doctors now" he said. "They are all here. Everyone is here and I will be just fine". I felt the hair on the back of my neck stand up. I knew that he was looking at people but it was not us. He kept repeating "I don't need no doctors now. They are all here". I turned to the students and told them that he was "*seeing Angel's*" now. It was an expression that I had begun to use after witnessing similar behavior in other patients. I have seen many people die. Most of them have no recall for the terminal event. It was a very solemn moment. I was very impressed. I had seen this behavior before, but never so intense. I commented that he would probably be dead in a few hours and he was, but he seemed physically fine at the time.

I have remembered that moment and his name all these years. It made an enormous impression on me. I know all the scientific explanations for such an event such as decreased blood flow to the brain, terminal neurons firing off, and many others. I am a man of science. I am spiritual, but not religious. I have no particular dogma or set of beliefs. I have attended many different churches through the years, from Catholic to Protestant. They never seemed to provide me with the spiritual knowledge that I was looking for. I really don't know what happened that day, but I think that this episode was something far beyond science. I was very emotionally moved. Perhaps, this is the realm of God.

Another day, while we were making rounds, a *"Code Blue"* was called on a patient down the hall. Code Blue, for those who don't know, means there is a critical patient whose heart and breathing have stopped. We do not run a Code Blue on patients who have a signed DNR (do not resuscitate) document with them. Other patients may be *in extremis*, but they are not technically a *Code Blue*. According to most of the information available, this means the brain has about 3 minutes to survive without permanent damage, unless the circulation is restored.

There was some mystery around this patient. He was a special patient in a bed reserved for infectious disease patients. He was separated from all the other patients, and only visited by infectious disease doctors. None of the regular house-staff had seen him. He was a special admission for the infectious disease doctors who were not yet in the hospital. So a Code had been called on this "mystery" patient and all the staff went pouring into the room.

I went to the head of the patient and started assisting ventilations with the Ambu bag. As I was trying to hold his head back, and chin up, his skin began to slough off in my hands. *This is not good*, I thought.

The woman performing chest compressions looked at me and asked "what is going on"? I told her that I didn't know, and nobody knew anything. He was a special Infectious Disease admission and we knew nothing about him. It did not look good. The patient expired and the Code was stopped.

Then someone from ID came into the room. All of us were told not to leave the room and to strip and surrender all our clothes to ID. This idea didn't go over very well with us. We all had a lot of work to do and, to be honest, I did not have many clothes. We did as we were told and stood around the room, naked, and feeling embarrassed for awhile. We were finally released from isolation after the ID folks had a meeting. We never found out what the patients diagnosis was, but there were a lot of guesses. Someone said cutaneous diphtheria, another said anthrax. We did not know and they never told us.

A usual day on the wards began with work rounds on the patients. Usually, this included the resident, two interns and the students. The case was discussed and a plan of action going forward was decided upon. All necessary tests were then ordered.

After this we would usually have Grand Rounds. This consisted of all the residents and interns, from the different services, meeting with the Chief of Medicine and other physician attendings. All new admissions were discussed and any problems on the wards were addressed.

When I became a resident, I would always instruct my interns not to mention any rashes that the patients may have. The reason for this was simple: We were never really sure why they had the rash and the differential diagnosis was extensive. The interns would present the new patient's case and let it be known that the patient indeed had a rash. The Chief of Medicine would then ask the intern what he thought the rash was caused by. The intern would usually claim ignorance. The Chief would then ask "well, who is your resident"? All eyes would then turn to me and ask the same question. I was usually thinking, *I told you not to mention the rash*, but it was too late.

So I would begin to rattle off a long list of possible causes and throw in a few exotic diseases for extra credit.

You know the old saying:" Baffle them with bullshit ". It is a lot like diplomacy in that "all options are on the table". This usually means that we have no definite idea what to do, but we will consider any and all options.

Another time, I learned the very real risks of responding to a Code Blue too quickly. The overhead intercom blared out that a Code Blue had been called in a room not far from where I was standing. I quickly ran down the hall and into the room. Remember, I was young, and this was a teaching hospital. In the room, there were 8 or 10 nurses and other hospital personnel present, but no doctor. Always, in other similar circumstances, there had been someone higher in the ranking than me. Not this time. All eyes turned to me for instruction. I turned around slowly and realized that I was the ranking individual this time. I thought, *Oops*! I began to give some orders. It was so strange watching people listen to me and following my lead. It was surreal. This patient actually responded well to the resuscitation efforts. I was ecstatic!

As the Code progressed, a surgical attending entered the room. I later overheard him comment to a nurse that it was one of the best run Codes that he had ever witnessed. *Good God*! I guess I was beginning to learn.

There was another incident, this time a painful lesson, that occurred while I was training. It involved a raphus tube. A raphus tube is an old device that was used by radiology to outline the duodenum (upper intestine). The raphus tube was a long, slender rubber hose attached to a football-shaped metal ball that measured about 1 inch long and ½ inches wide. The metal ball had slits along its sides. The idea was to place the metal ball in the duodenum and then inject some contrast dye to facilitate visualization. Well, I was the intern and he was my patient.

Radiology sent the raphus tube upstairs to me and asked that it be placed in the patient before sending him down for the study. I had never seen or heard of the tube, so I asked my resident how to place it. He replied that he wasn't sure, but it probably went down the nose, and into the stomach like a naso-gastric tube that we placed all the time. I said "OK" and went to the patient with the tube and explained what we needed to do for the study. He just accepted the necessity and agreed to allow the procedure.

He had more trust in me than I deserved. I proceeded to hold his head back, as you would for an NG tube, and tried to insert the metal ball into his nostril. Fortunately, he had large nostrils because the metal ball was pretty big. Well, I tried and tried, but the ball would not fit. Soon the patient was squirming, and shifting back in the chair as far as he could go. Tears began to roll down his cheeks, but I was very determined to be a good intern and do my job. By now, he was writhing in pain and tossing his head back and forth, but I kept going. Finally, the large metal ball slipped through his nares and into his throat. The patient had had enough. He reached up, grabbed the rubber tube and yanked the metal ball out of his nose.

His nose began to bleed profusely, but I did not let that stop me. I held pressure on that nostril to stop the bleeding and explained quickly that it was alright, he had another nostril. I proceeded to climb into the chair and straddle him. I stuffed the metal ball into the other nostril.

By now, the patient was yelling and writhing, but I kept shoving. Finally, we succeeded in getting the metal ball through his nose, down his throat and into his stomach. I taped the tube to the side of his nose, wiped the sweat off my brow, and sent him down to radiology for the study.

Soon after he arrived in radiology, one of the radiologists called to the floor and wanted to know who the "idiot" was that had put the raphus tube down his nose. Apparently, patients were simply supposed to swallow the device. I admitted my guilt and could not believe what I had done. *Oh Lord*, I thought, *I have put this man through so much pain and discomfort.*

Patients are just too willing to accept whatever a doctor tells them. Doctors don't always know what is right, and I was only an intern. In my defense, I had asked my resident and he did not know either. Whenever there is a question, the resident is the person to go to. If they don't know, they can usually find out.

While I was at the VA, on general medicine again, I had a bad COPD patient. He was an older gentleman who simply could not breathe well. COPD stands for chronic obstructive pulmonary disease. Most cases, but not all, are related to chronic smoking as his was. It was all new then, but of course, I found out later that it is a very common diagnosis. We gave him the usual treatment of inhaled bronchodilators and IV steroids.

He was getting better, so I was very surprised to arrive one morning and find out that he had died during the night. I hung my head and started out of the room, when one of his roommates cried out "don't feel bad Doc. After each breathing treatment, he would feel better and go out to smoke cigarettes". I still felt bad, but it helped to know that I had been doing the right stuff. You can't fight City Hall or a smoking addiction. I also had many diabetic patients, who would sit in the hall and cheat on their diabetic diets by eating candy bars. As the saying goes:"You can lead a horse to water, but you can't make him drink".

Another episode involved a very sick man with bilateral (both sides) pneumonia. In the real world, this man was so ill that he would have been placed in a bed, at rest, with oxygen and IV antibiotics. This was not the real world. It was an academic institution. Therefore, we had to sit him up, run a tube into his lungs, aspirate (suck out) some of the fluid and make a gram stain slide. This was all for morning rounds the next day. During this procedure he suffered a Code Blue and died. I was so angry. It seemed so unnecessary, so academic, but that was the way it was then. I could not wait to get out of academic medicine.

I finally entered the last two months of my Residency. They announced the attending physicians for all the rotations, and I drew Dr. "Mean Joe" Griffith. They did not call him "Mean Joe" for nothing. He had a reputation for being gruff and unapproachable. I wasn't scared, but I thought, *Christ, what bad luck*! The first few days were a bit rocky as everyone was "feeling" each other out.

Eventually, I found out that Dr. "Mean Joe" was great. He had learned to avoid many common hassles such as harassing "hall consultations". In a "hall consultation", other physicians would stop the physician and simply ask for their opinion. He wasn't really mean at all. He was smart, efficient, and accessible, and he would go to the "mat" to protect any of his house-staff, if he thought they were right. It turned out to be a wonderful learning experience, and he was truly one of the best attendings that I ever had the pleasure to know.

I only received one negative comment from all my attendings (intructors) on the various rotations. The attendings usually grade and make comments on each student, after the rotation. A pulmonary medicine attending stated that I did not have enough patience to be a good internist. I hate to admit it, but he was right. I am not gifted with an abundance of patience. I suppose that is another reason that I chose to pursue the practice of Emergency Medicine. In this specialty, the physician can practice both medicine and minor surgery, without immersing themselves completely in either specialty. It really fit my personality. *See them and street them,* as they say. In actuality, the patient is seen, the diagnosis is made, the patient is stabilized or the treatment is begun, and then their care is transferred to another physician, or they are discharged. This is the essence of Emergency Medicine.

CHAPTER 4

The Veteran's Administration

THE VETERAN'S ADMINISTRATION SET UP A hospital system, that is separate from the private hospital system, to provide lifetime healthcare for all of the existing veterans. It is a noble concept.

However, in my opinion, the Veteran's Administration (now called the Department of Veterans Affairs) is an example of a good idea gone wrong. I worked at the VA during the late 1970's and 80's, and have dealt with the system many times as a private emergency physician. I feel that this experience has qualified me to express my opinion of the system.

I do not feel that a completely separate system of health care delivery for veterans is necessary and here is why. The VA system is fantastic for post-amputee rehabilitation, as well as other combat-related trauma victims. However, in my experience, easily 80% of the inpatient VA hospital care was for hypertension, diabetes, heart-related issues and the ubiquitous alcohol abuse related medical issues. These types of medical issues are easily provided for in the existing public hospital system. This would have the added benefit of trimming the hospital staff needed for a separate hospital system such as nurses, lab techs, x-ray techs and more. VA medical facilities have federal employees, who are compensated at a significantly higher rate than similar private employees. In my experience, they often do not perform as well as the private employees.

In addition, the veterans themselves would no longer have to drive 3 or 4 hours to sit in a VA clinic every few months to get their problems checked and a new prescription, if necessary. They could simply see their local physician, whom they would know, and present a certified VA card for the government to pay their health expenses as they were promised. If they needed an admission, they would have the option of staying at their local hospital; this would facilitate family visits. Again, the expense could be billed through their certified VA card and the government would then assume the debt as promised to the veteran. This would essentially work like Medicare or most private insurance policies. It might even result in superior care and cost saving, while fulfilling the obligation to the veteran.

The current system—or at least the one in effect when I worked at the VA— all too often, results in the veteran being transported by ambulance from their home and stopping at a local hospital for temporary stabilization. Then, by law, the emergency physician has to call ahead to the receiving VA hospital and obtain permission for transport and acceptance. All too often, the receiving VA will neither accept nor deny transport. This action relieves them from any financial liability, but leaves the veteran lying in some strange, uncomfortable ER bed for hours or even days. Only when the VA accepts or denies transfer, will the government accept responsibility for the veteran's medical bill. If their problem becomes acute, then the local physician will admit the patient and provide the necessary medical or surgical treatment, knowing that now the VA system will never compensate them for this. In this manner, the VA avoids financial responsibility for the veteran's medical care. This is unacceptable. I, personally, have advocated for an ailing veteran by phoning a senator early in the morning, to get him to place a call to the local VA hospital and have them perform their job. This was after the veteran had spent several days in my ER. If they would just deny the transport, then the local physician would have some chance of future compensation. The problem has become so severe that I would instruct the paramedics not to stop at any outlying hospital, unless they were concerned about the immediate health of the veteran. Once they stop, the VA will never accept or deny the transport. The veterans have no idea that they are being treated so callously.

Even when veterans actually accessed a VA facility, however, they sometimes would face a frustrating runaround. A case that I recall involved a veteran who had a local private doctor and ordinarily would never come to the VA. His non-VA doctor was out of town and he needed his blood pressure medicine refilled. He had come to the hospital that morning, and I encountered him late in the afternoon in the cardiology clinic. He had spent all day being sent from one clinic to the next because no one would listen to his story or accept responsibility for refilling his prescription. He was so frustrated by the time I saw him that he was actually crying. He sobbed that he just wanted his blood pressure medicine.

I gave him the medicine and told him never to come back. He agreed, thanked me, and ran out of the hospital.

I have many such VA horror stories. Perhaps it has all been fixed and the system is much better now, but I doubt it. These are some of the cases that I observed while working at the VA.

I was an intern assigned to general medicine at the local VA hospital. All of the patients who are admitted to the hospital are evaluated by the Admitting Officer of the Day (AOD), and then assigned to a particular service, depending on their health problem. The AOD is a doctor who works for the VA system. The house-staff, who run the services, work for the teaching hospital. By the rules of the VA hospital system, the house-staff are not allowed to communicate with the AOD. This is important because of what happened next.

I was working on general medicine when I was informed of an admission to my service from the AOD. The working diagnosis was given as "unobtainable blood pressure- please admit to general medicine". I went over to the patient to begin my exam and evaluation. I was shocked to discover that the patient was, in fact, dead. All I could think was, *My God, no wonder they could not get a blood pressure- he is dead!* This was truly unbelievable. A man with medical training had admitted a dead man to the hospital. I knew that I was not supposed to discuss any cases with a VA doctor, but I was so enraged at this ridiculous situation that I ran down the stairs to the AOD's office and began to loudly discuss how inappropriate I found this particular admission. All he had to say in his defense was that it was almost 5 PM on a Friday afternoon and he was trying to clear all the patients from his department.

I was appalled. Admittedly, I had not been a doctor for very long, but I had never seen or expected to see such callous disregard for human life. This man had a family, a wife and children that had no idea what was happening. I found the wife and tried to explain the incredibly sad facts to her. I then went and admitted the dead man to my service as required by the rules. I immediately pronounced him dead, and filled out the required forms for this. I kept thinking, *this is totally insane.*

Another episode involved a rural gentleman. He was a good man who had a terrible diagnosis. He worked a farm just south of town. His wife had come to the VA hospital with him. I had admitted him to Intensive Care while I tried to prove the suspected diagnosis. I thought he suffered from a disease called bacterial endocarditis. This is basically an infection of the heart valves. It isn't common, and is very hard to diagnose. Unfortunately, the patient can dissolve the heart valve and die. It was this outcome that I was trying to avoid.

The technology at that time was limited, so visualizing the valves and proving the diagnosis was extremely difficult. Most patients will require a mechanical valve if the heart valve erodes. The heart surgeons were understandably reluctant to operate on the patient without more evidence of the diagnosis.

I had admitted him to Intensive Care because of his suspected, but not proven diagnosis. In this setting the nurses have one patient for their entire shift. It is referred to as a one-on-one situation.

When I would arrive to examine the patient or just talk, I would often find his nurse with her feet propped up on the counter and reading a magazine. I asked her if she knew what his vital signs were or the latest temperature. She did not know anything. I inquired about the food spilled on his chest and she replied that she was going to "train" him not to spill his food while eating. Of course, he only spilled his food because he was so ill. His wife had even pleaded to be allowed in and help him with his food, but the nurse had not allowed this. I became enraged and asked her if she even knew what bacterial endocarditis was and therefore what his prognosis (outcome) might be. She had no idea. This man died a few days later and the autopsy confirmed my suspicion, but it was too late to help him.

I was called to the Medical Office to explain my behavior. I was informed that the nurses work for the VA, and I had no business trying to make her do her job. I tried to defend myself by explaining that I had worked at several other non-VA hospitals and I had found the nurses to be very competent and willing to work. They dismissed my argument. I had many visits to the Medical Office, for verbal reprimands, during my tenure at the VA.

I had another outrageous experience at the VA. The patient was an elderly male who was a very difficult "stick". This means that when drawing blood or starting an IV, it is very difficult for medical staff to locate and access a suitable vein near the patient's skin.

The usual routine at this hospital was for the lab tech or phlebotomist to acquire the blood for testing in the morning. By early afternoon the results would appear on the chart. If the lab did not process the blood during the

AM run, the entire process would be repeated again the next day. If at any time there were any problems getting the blood, then supposedly the tech would notify the doctor (me) and let him try to get it.

The system failed two days in a row. I would review the chart in the afternoon looking for the lab-work, but it wasn't there. Upon following the trail of possible errors, I discovered that the blood had never been drawn. To make matters worse, I discovered that the tech had never even tried to get the blood. They would stand at the door, according to the patient, and never come in or try to obtain any blood. Then, they would fail to notify anyone of the failure to obtain blood, so of course, in the afternoon, there would be no results. I was furious.

The next day, events began to unfold as they had the previous days. This time I was ready. After determining that no blood had been drawn, I drew it myself (which involved several painful sticks for the patient), then hand-carried the blood to the lab with the appropriate orders.

The tech was busy reading a magazine when I came into the lab. I signed the blood into the register as required and explained to the tech how difficult it had been to acquire this blood. It had now been several days and the lab results were very important. I explained to him how difficult it had been to obtain the blood and how important the results were. He nodded in agreement and took the blood tubes. I then proceeded to leave the lab, but happened to look back as the lab door closed.

The door had a glass window in it and I watched as the lab tech took the tubes of blood and threw them in the trash and went back to his magazine. I was enraged.

The blood had been so hard to obtain, and the patient had undergone multiple painful sticks for this. I ran back upstairs and started trying to track down the head of the laboratory by phone. After several attempts, I found him at a local restaurant. I quickly told him what had happened and strongly urged him to make his lab tech get the blood tubes out of the trash and get the lab results. He did, and the lab results were obtained at last. Of course, after this exchange, I was called to the Medical Office—again.

On another occasion at the VA, earlier in my career, I was a student on general surgery. We had a patient who had a terrible problem. He had cancer of the mouth and was going to require extensive surgery and radiation therapy. He would require removal of the mandible (jawbone) and a bilateral (both sides) radical neck dissection. We discussed the operative procedure with him and the severity of his disease process. He agreed with the decision for surgery.

The plan was that during the surgery, after the removal of the patient's mandible, a flap of skin would be cut from the patient's chest and transferred to his mouth to repair it. Thus, before the main operation, a doctor marked off the target area on the patient's chest and made some preliminary incisions in the skin. This would facilitate the removal of the skin flap later when it was needed. Everything went as planned, and the patient was prepped for surgery. The day of the surgery arrived. The attending physician was to be assisted by the chief resident. I would be present to provide any extra help that might be needed. The surgery began, and I was observing with fascination.

After about one hour, the attending "broke scrub" and left the operating room. This left me and the chief resident (who by definition is still in training) to perform an extensive operation. The operating room nurses witnessed as things began to go wrong.

The radical neck dissection to remove any lymph nodes resulted in a lot of bleeding, but we gained control and continued on. I was getting worried, but felt that as a student I should keep my mouth shut. Then we discovered that the incisions on the upper chest, for the skin flap that was needed, had been placed too low were of no use. The chief resident forged ahead, creating a flap of skin from the top of his shaved head. This was swung down to make the floor of the mouth. The moved flap of skin had a tenuous blood supply and we almost lost it; but we managed to save it and make it work. A drawback was that now he would have hair growing in his mouth the rest of his life, if he survived.

There was so much blood oozing from the patient. We finished the operation and repaired all the wounds.

When we had finished, and I thought about what we had done to that man, I could not help wondering if surgery had been the right choice. He had a large incision on his chest and his new mouth would grow hair in it. It was then that I learned the attending had left to take care of some "personal business". This type of behavior would never be tolerated in a public hospital, and it should not be tolerated in the VA. The patient survived his surgery, only to die from his cancer a few months later.

In my opinion, the VA system manages conflict trauma and rehabilitation very well. The contract that exists between our government and the veterans for lifetime health benefits is a noble and just endeavor that should be honored. However, it seems to me, as I stated before, that providing the veteran with a government card and then allowing them to redeem the health benefits at their local doctor or hospital might result in a better health care experience for the veterans. In addition, it would most likely be much more convenient for their families should they require hospitalization. The government would then assume their health costs, thereby honoring the contract. There would be no need for long trips for the veteran, to sit in a clinic and see a strange doctor, just for a routine check and prescription. There would be no need for duplicate hospital systems with the needed ancillary services such as radiology and laboratory. I see no benefit in a separate and difficult to reach health care delivery system.

This would probably result in cost savings, in a time of increasing austerity, while providing health care for the veterans as promised. The current system also results in all of the hospital employee's becoming federal employee's and compensated at a significantly higher rate than similar private employees. It is truly sad to see a veteran who begins to realize that the "lifetime health benefits" that they were promised, and rightfully expected, have significant "strings" attached.

CHAPTER 5

The Real World—from Academics to Real World Medicine

I FINALLY COMPLETED MY INTERNSHIP WHICH was sufficient for me to apply for and obtain my license to practice medicine. Due to financial difficulties, I did not pursue further education in a specialty, which would have required serving for several more years in a hospital as a low-paid resident doctor. I quit academics and went to work in the emergency department. The financial difficulties were simply that I ran out of money and my family would not help. The salary paid to an intern or resident is adequate, but meager. It was a common practice in those days to go to work in an ER in order to boost the salary, but fortunately for the patients, not anymore.

I took a job on the coast of North Carolina and went to work. The first few shifts went well with no major problems. I remember being very surprised at the incredibly deferential and respectful attitudes that these nurses had for me as a doctor. I was not accustomed to that from my years in academia, and it felt wrong to be treated so differently from anyone else.

On one of the first shifts I worked, I entered the staff lounge to introduce myself, and all the nurses stood up to give me their chair. I looked around to see if someone had come in behind me. It finally dawned on me that this was their usual behavior and I assured everyone that I was not like that and asked them to please sit back down. It made me feel very uncomfortable to be treated like royalty. We all got along fine as we got to know each other and began to relax. In talking with the staff, it became apparent that some doctors expected to be treated like kings.

It was probably the third shift when things changed radically. The ambulance called in to announce the impending arrival of a young girl with multiple injuries from an auto accident. In most instances, there is only one patient in each ambulance. It seems that two cars, with two teenage girls in each, had been racing after school when they hit a bridge and crashed. Eventually we found out that the emergency medical technicians (EMT's) were bringing in not just one, but all four girls. On arrival, the first girl was dead, the second girl had multiple fractures and a ruptured spleen, the third girl had a punctured lung and scalp lacerations, and the fourth girl had only contusions and a few lacerations. I was extremely excited, almost panicky. I was not trained for this. I could put in a few stitches, but I knew medicine, not trauma.

I switched into "automatic" and began to work on the three arriving patients who had survived. I got all the bleeding stopped, put them all on oxygen, restored blood pressures with intravenous fluids and stabilized the fractures. I spoke on the phone with the "doc" at the receiving hospital, to let him know what was coming. He suggested that I place a chest tube in the girl with the punctured lung. A chest tube is used to drain blood or air from the lung space in the chest. I replied that I had never done this procedure and he began to explain the details over the phone. So I began. I identified the rib space on her side that I would use, injected the area with lidocaine to "numb" it, and then I made the skin incision. I inserted the Kelly clamp (a large curved metal clamp) spread all the connective tissue and muscle by opening the Kelly very wide and making the "hole" larger. Then, I pushed the Kelly clamp forward in order to push through the pleura (lining of the lung). I felt it "pop" as I entered the lung space. I inserted a finger into the hole to feel for lung tissue and then inserted the plastic chest tube. I sewed it in place and secured it with tape and a bandage, then hooked it to a Pleur-evac collection chamber (a plastic container for blood, air and fluid) and hooked it to wall suction. I was extremely nervous. I had never made a hole in someone's chest before.

Eventually, I had stabilized all the patients and had begun to ship them to the receiving hospital. There, we expected, they could receive definitive care for their problems. I remember feeling very tired as the last ambulance pulled away on its way to the larger hospital.

A few minutes went by, and the radio came to life again. The last ambulance to depart had made it to the county line when it wrecked, and now the new victims were coming in. The young girl had new fractures and the ambulance driver just had some fractures and a few lacerations. I repaired the lacerations and stabilized the fractures, but now we had to use one of the old hearses for transport because we were out of ambulances.

The rest of the shift was relatively uneventful. *Thank God*, I thought.

There was a nurse, by the name of Helen, working in this emergency department. Helen was very outgoing and a pleasure to work with. In addition to being a great ER nurse, she had a fun personality and knew most everyone. She was young, pretty, and had dated most of the local cops and highway patrol. This came in handy for me one day when I was pulled over by one of the highway patrolmen. We started talking, and when he found out that I knew Helen he decided against giving me a ticket and just laughed and waved me on.

I remember another incident that involved Helen. A young male trauma victim was brought into the ER by EMS. He had a very large bulge in his groin and I noticed Helen staring at it. According to trauma protocols, we had to remove all his clothes anyway, so I laughed at Helen and told her to go ahead and take his pants off. Faster than lightening his pants were removed and the look of disappointment on her face was far larger than his "bulge". It turned out to be a bag of marijuana that he had taped to his thigh to avoid the cops. I heard her disillusionment as she commented – "I knew nobody was "hung" so well". Fortunately, his injuries were minor but her disappointment was major. We all laughed and joked at her expense. As we often did when we found drugs on a patient, we just threw it away.

There was another incident, much later, that occurred in which the ER staff again found a "stash" on a trauma patient. This time it turned out to be a large wad of hundred dollar bills. The victim was unconscious, and therefore unable to explain the cash. A few hours later, two very large males showed up, asking about the money. They did not seem to be very interested in the victims' health status. We denied any knowledge of the cash and told them it must have been in his car. I have found over the years that it is best to stay out of certain situations, if you can. We just turned the money over to the police. It really wasn't our problem.

On another shift, I saw something that I had never seen before and hope I never see again. It was my first burn victim. Burn patients are not particularly difficult to treat, but they are extremely hard to witness. It was mid-winter and cold outside. It seems that some mother had left her children at home alone and they were trying to build a fire in the fireplace to stay warm. A three year old boy had set himself aflame while trying to make the fire.

The ambulance announced their pending arrival. On arrival, the boy was stable, but he had sustained third-degree burns (severe) from his waist up. He never spoke, complained, or moved. His airway was in jeopardy from swelling, so I had to intubate him. I will always remember his sad, scared eyes looking up at me. He was just a little boy, surrounded by strangers and in terrific pain. He was very afraid. We could not find the parents. We knew his chances for survival were very small, but we did our job and got him stabilized with fluids and pain meds. Then we transferred him to the Burn Clinic in Chapel Hill. I found out later that he died.

I recall another situation at this hospital. Remember, this all took place more than three decades ago. We still had assistants called orderlies in those days. The young man working as an orderly in the ER happened to be black. This was rural North Carolina and race relations were not incredibly enlightened to say the least. In fact, I suspect that the KKK was still alive and well there. The orderly's name was Sam. Sam was young, fun and very outgoing. We became good friends.

We were working in the ER one night when an older white woman drove her husband up to the ER entrance. Sam went out to the car with a wheel-chair, to assist the gentleman, as his wife watched. He turned out to be very drunk. The ER was accessed through a set of double glass sliding doors with a space between them. Sam helped the man out of the car and into the chair and started into the ER. They were in this small space between the sliding doors when the man woke up, looked around, then yelled to his wife "Oh Martha, there's a n***** in here".

Sam stopped pushing the chair and began to dance around while shouting "where, where". He then hit the button to open the doors and lunged out of the space. We were all just rolling with laughter at the scene. It was wonderfully funny and nobody was hurt. Sam always insisted that he wasn't black, but that he was Jamaican. He was a good friend.

Another time, a little old lady, with wild white hair poking out from under a cap, came into the ER because of a lower leg laceration. As I was sewing up the cut, I asked her how this had happened. She explained that while she was splitting some wood for the fire, a piece had flown over and struck her in the leg. This wonderful old lady must have been in her mid-ninety's. All I could think was that I hoped I could still split wood at ninety!

Another episode involved an older, retired couple. It was early in the morning and they had been working a paper route when he developed chest pain. After talking with them, it became apparent that they had been together for a very long time and knew each other well. Unfortunately for him, the work-up revealed that he was indeed having a very large heart attack. He already had some signs of heart failure, so that made his chances of dying very high.

They looked at each other for a long while and held hands. Then she said "goodbye", and that she would be back later, after she finished the paper route. I had such mixed emotions. I was incredibly sad, but I was so amazed by their love for each other. I hoped that one day; I could also have such a wonderful relationship. I was stunned for a moment. I never saw them again.

Another incident involved a "working girl". The lady was well known to the local police force and was working one evening, when a couple of officers arrested her again. They were on their way to jail when apparently some sort of deal was reached. They drove off into the woods to work out the terms of the agreement. The officers were apparently distracted by the anticipated amorous events and accidently hit the transmit button on their radio. The entire county listened as they moaned and groaned during their incidental tryst. In the ER, we received a frantic call from the jail as they searched for the amorous officers. They never found them. The officers strolled into the headquarters, after the encounter, and were greeted by an enraged captain. Apparently their behavior was unappreciated.

Another episode involved ER security. A patient was checking in at triage, when he became agitated, pulled out a knife, jumped over the counter, and took the secretary hostage. The police were already in the ER, because they would hang out at night and flirt with the nurses. I learned that in a lot of small towns, the only place open in the wee hours of the morning was the ER. They would often pitch in and help with any belligerent patients. I was glad to have them. They surrounded the man with knife, tried to get him to surrender, then finally, one of the officers shot the man. He was dead.

Security in the ER is a huge and growing problem. I have seen gun battles, hostages, and stabbings. In fact, I have been in several altercations myself. Patients, or their friends, are often very angry with the ER staff for a variety of reasons. Maybe they did not get the meds they wanted, or they thought had waited too long, or they did not like the diagnosis. There are usually no armed guards and the patients often have weapons. I began to carry a "stun" gun to work for protection. Some ER's now have secure access to the department and maybe this will help. I am not sure what can be done, but I don't care to have my nurses or myself threatened with violence.

The personalities of the doctors' on-call at each ER are different, as anticipated. There were a couple of physicians at this ER that stood out. One of them was a gentleman who taught me the value of good salesmanship. He would often tell the relatives that he had "stopped the pus just before it got to the heart". It was great. Of course, it was a lie, but it was a great lie. In these cases there was never any pus— the relative often had a very mild viral illness— but all the relatives and friends thought he was magnificent. The relatives did not know any medicine and no harm was done. As they say in sports *"no harm, no foul"*.

I continued to work in that ER for another year and learned a great deal. The nurses were very kind to me. If I was late for a shift, they would send the cops by my house. They knew that I often had car trouble, and that I would be walking to work. The cops would find me and give me a ride to the ER. The nurses knew that I loved the mountains and offered to "build" me a mountain in the North Carolina swamps if I would just stay, but I could not. I wanted to be in the mountains and kept taking jobs that got me closer and closer.

I rented a cabin in Asheville, on the banks of the French Broad River. It was spectacular. I felt I had "died and gone to heaven". I was young and incredibly naïve, but I was finally in the mountains. I loved to backpack and would often head over to the Shining Rock area, and even hiked Cold Mountain. A novel written by Charles Frazier refers to Cold Mountain. I suppose that is one of the reasons that I enjoyed the book so much. I lived in Asheville and worked a number of nearby hospitals.

I was working at another ER, near Charlotte, one day when a man came in who had snagged his right eye with a treble-hook while fishing. It was a very bad injury and I found an ophthalmologist to care for it. The patient had a family physician, but he needed an ophthalmologist for this injury. No general doctor, in his or her right mind treats complicated eye problems. We just don't have the training.

This man's family doctor found out that I had arranged for an ophthalmologist to see the guy. The doctor came down to the ER to "cuss" me out for not calling him. I shouted back that he just wanted to get the extra charge on the chart. He would never or should never try to fix that kind of injury himself.

It was at this ER that I caught an ER nurse reading the x-ray's and treating patients on her own. She would not even notify me that there was a patient in the ED that needed to be seen. Many emergency departments had a small office or an on-call room that the doctor could go to in between patients. I was in the on-call room and left it to go wandering around the ED. I discovered her treating an actively seizing patient one day. She had never tried to notify me that there was a patient in the ED. For the patient, this can be a dangerous situation. I knew that this behavior was a hold-over from prior years when there was no doctor available in the ED, but times had changed.

After an intense verbal battle, I told her that this kind of behavior would not be tolerated when I was working. After all, my name was all over the charts and if any thing should go wrong, I would get the blame. The hospital would not address the problem of such nurses and the ER company that controlled the ER activities did not particularly care. I discovered how little weight my opinion carried. I refused to go back to that hospital.

Here is a brief explanation of how ER staffing works. There are two basic types of emergency department practice. In my opinion, having worked in both types, the best is the private ED group. In the private situation, a group of ED physician's band together, and agree to provide coverage to a specific hospital. The staff physicians learn the ED doctors and vice-versa.

The other situation is a large contract group. This type of organization typically enters into contracts with many emergency departments and promise to provide their coverage. They then recruit a number of physician's and plug them into the emergency departments where they need them. These contract groups often have one or two full-time ER doc's and many part-time physicians with a variety of backgrounds. Of course, the physician has to acquire hospital privileges in order to work at a particular hospital. In my opinion, this is less than ideal for a variety of reasons, but this is the current system.

I was working in another emergency department, when some of the staff and I went out to a local bar for some fun. The county this hospital was in was a "dry" county but we found a bar on the county line. It was a real dump with windows at ground level, cinder-block construction, and patrons urinating through the windows into the bar. But it was open, so we went in and grabbed a booth. We got some beer and began swapping stories.

About that time, a very large "gentleman" walked into the bar. He looked like he had just stepped off of a Harley-Davidson motorcycle. He had a .45 pistol on one hip and a large knife on the other. He had multiple tattoos and long, greasy hair. One of the guys at our table began to shout at him "Hey, Fat-Ass". We all sank lower in our seats. The large man did not turn around, so our friend yelled out again "Hey, Fat-Ass, I'm talking to you". All I could think was that we were all about to die and I didn't even know these people very well.

The large man began to slowly turn around and I could just barely make out his face through all the cigarette smoke and dim light. He looked over at our table, and I shifted further down in the seat. He walked toward us. Then his face lit up with a big toothless grin and he shouted "hello" to the guy at our table. He started laughing and grabbed the guy in a big bear-hug. It turns out that they knew each other and his nickname really was "Fat-Ass". His brother "Nasty" was still outside with the bikes. I was incredibly relieved.

I was working another emergency department, near Asheville, when I had a patient encounter that would lead to my first malpractice case. It was late at night and the shift had been difficult. An older woman came in to the department for abdominal pain. She had been driven in by her family. On examination, she did not appear to be in any acute distress and her vital signs were all normal. Her abdomen was mildly tender to deep palpation, but there was no evidence of increased tympany or rebound tenderness (these are physical findings that suggest intestinal or stomach perforation, or distended bowel). By auscultation (listening with a stethoscope) the bowel sounds were normal. Her lab tests were fine, showing a normal white blood count and hemoglobin, as well as normal chemistries. A urinalysis was also done and it too appeared normal.

At this point, it seemed that this was an elderly female with a mild stomach ache, but no fever and a normal blood pressure. I did not obtain any diagnostic x-rays because they did not appear to be needed. Moreover, in those days the radiology technician did not stay in the hospital and would have to be called back in. This proved to be a large mistake on my part.

I telephoned her local physician, who happened to be on-call, and explained the case to him. At that point, I thought she may have a stomach ulcer and I was trying to have her admitted for treatment and further diagnostic testing. I did not feel that she was in distress at all. Her doctor said he knew the patient well and she was always complaining about something. Now, I made my next big mistake: I believed him. He again assured me that he knew her very well and that I should "just give her something for pain" and he would see her in the morning in the office. I did what he suggested, but then kept her in the ED for observation for a few hours. I did not like to give pain medicine to a patient with undiagnosed abdominal pain.

She remained stable and her pain subsided, so I discharged her with instructions to see her local physician in the morning in the office. She did not go to the office in the morning.

My shift ran until late that afternoon and she came rolling in by ambulance at about four PM. Now, she was obviously in distress with perforated bowel (it was found to be a perforated duodenal ulcer, which is the same as bowel, at surgery). According to the daughter, at about noon, she complained of acute mid-abdominal pain, turned pale, and fell back in the bed. The family continued to watch her until late afternoon, then called an ambulance. I would have thought that they would call for an ambulance when her symptoms changed. She had failed to follow-up in the morning with her local doctor and that was regrettable.

The woman went straight to the operating room, where the surgeon found a perforated stomach(duodenal) ulcer. Unfortunately, now it was far too late and the woman died.

It was of little consolation, but I had been right about the stomach ulcer.

Afterward, her local doctor said that he thought I had been talking about another patient of his and had he been aware, of course he would have admitted her. I learned the hard way about "telephone consultations".

My attorney explained that since I had not obtained an x-ray of her abdomen that I would lose the case. I tried to defend myself by producing large volumes of literature, from respectable medical journals, that spoke of the indications for an x-ray, and that my patient had no indications. The attorney explained that the literature would just "confuse the jury" and that the telephone consult was useless.

I spent three years feeling terrible, angry, depressed and convinced that I was a very poor physician. I had volumes of respectable medical literature to back me up, the worthless testimony of a confused local physician, repeated physical exams, and a willingness by the patient to follow-up with her physician in the morning, but I did not have an x-ray. My attorney explained that lay-people believe that x-rays are "magic", regardless of what they show. In the end, they asked for one million dollars in compensation and settled for thirty-five thousand dollars.

I was young and did not know what a game malpractice suits had become. I thought to myself that if the family truly believed that I had killed their mother, then why did they settle? Surely their mother was worth more than thirty-five thousand dollars. I learned to my astonishment that in a malpractice case, there is no "trial by a jury of your peers" as guaranteed in the constitution. It was not the fault of the jury. They had no medical training and simply had to believe what they were told. The prosecution hired "expert witnesses" who all explained that you had handled the case all wrong. The defense hired "expert witnesses" who all explained that you did everything right. The jury did not know. It appeared that whoever put on the "best show" would win the case. I thought it was supposed to be about *the truth*. How silly is that?

I was disillusioned with EM and I had broken-up with my girlfriend, so I left Asheville. We had been together for a few years, but it wasn't working out, so I left. I began working an ED near Statesville, and lived in a room in the old Nurse's Dormitory right beside the hospital. This worked well since my car was broken and it kept the walking down to a minimum.

Money was tight, as usual. The arrangement worked well during the week, but I had to vacate the room on the weekends to allow the part-time doctors to use it for a call-room. I would just hitch-hike to Charlotte, make a run of the bars, and hopefully find a lady who would let me stay with her for the weekend. Then I would hitch back to the hospital and move back into the dorm room for the week. One day, on a return trip to the hospital, I had to walk in from the interstate with a full 45 pound pack. It was hot, humid and I was sweating like a mule. I was hitching the entire distance, when one of the nurses from the hospital passed me, continued on and waved. When I ran into her, later at the hospital, I inquired as to why she had just passed me on the road and not given me a ride? She explained that she thought I was "practicing backpacking". It was well known that I truly enjoyed backpacking, but I couldn't help thinking that you don't really have to practice walking. She meant well, she just didn't know.

In this ER, there were a couple of regular patients that I can recall. The first one was a man named John. John was in his mid-fifties and was a Vietnam Veteran. He had a real bad habit of getting drunk and then coming to the ER. John was a belligerent, angry drunk, but he was usually fairly easy to deal with if someone would just listen to him. I had a lot of experience from my childhood in dealing with "drunks"; my mother had been a heavy drinker. Unfortunately, a male nurse who worked there felt it necessary to go into the room and aggravate John. Then, John would explode, tear up the room, turn the bed over, bend the IV poles and threaten anyone who came near him.

It was all so unnecessary. Several times I asked this nurse why he had to aggravate John? Why not just listen to him, treat his complaint and move on? He never really gave me an answer. Usually, I could work with John, calm him down, and send him on his way. Sometimes, it would not work, and we would have to call the cops. It is hard to run an ED with someone screaming and tossing furniture around.

The other regular patient was a mid-forties female who would show up every few weeks for an anti-anxiety shot. She was pretty harmless, raising children on her own and working. Periodically, she would just get overwhelmed with life and all its problems and come to the ER. She could be fairly dramatic about it all. She was a big woman and once lay on the floor off the waiting room as if she had passed out. I went out to make sure that she was alright and that the unconsciousness was not real. Having done so, I told her that I could not pick her up and when she felt better, she could come on back.

I suspect that the other patients in the waiting room felt that this was a cold approach, but I had known this woman for months and I did not have the personnel to waste on a fake fainting attack. In a few moments, she pulled herself together and came on back for treatment. I listened to her talk about her hard life and how no-one helped and it was "just too much". I gave her the anti-anxiety shot, she felt better, went home and made it for another few weeks.

Another time, a woman drove her husband to the local doctor's office. He was having chest pain, but unfortunately by the time they arrived, he was dead in the front seat of the car. The doctor examined him in the car, determined he was dead, and told the woman to "drive straight to the ER". He then called me, in the ED, to let me know that a patient was coming and that he was probably dead. Incredulously, I asked if anyone was performing CPR on the patient and he just replied "no". This poor woman was driving her dead husband across town and hoping we could save him. I wish I had something to offer her.

Another episode caught my attention. A couple's small child had banged her forehead on some furniture and sustained a very small laceration to the right forehead. If I had been a parent, had I seen this at home I would have placed a band-aid or maybe some steri-strips, and let it go. Instead, the parents stood by her side, and the local doctor. They had even called in the local surgeon for a repair. Obviously, they were well-connected and heavily insured. Meanwhile, I was struggling to repair a large, irregular chain-saw laceration on another gentleman's face. He really did need someone with better surgical skills than me, but he had little money and no insurance, so it was me or nobody. It was another lesson in the double-standards in medicine.

I had several dealings with that surgeon, but one circumstance from many years ago stands out. A young man presented to the ER after a car accident. He was in bad shape with his blood pressure dropping. Remember, this was many years ago. I knew the boy needed a blood transfusion, or he would not make the journey, by ambulance, to the receiving hospital. I tried desperately to get a central line going, both in the subclavian vein and in the internal carotid vein. His peripheral veins were all collapsed due to blood loss and resulting hypotension.

I had no luck obtaining a central line and requested help from the surgeon. He refused to help. Instead, he suggested that I just toss the patient in the ambulance as he was and send him to Charlotte. I was furious.

This occurred before COBRA or EMTALA, which are laws that were passed to prevent the transfer of unstable patients and usually poor or uninsured patients. Now the patients have to have a physical exam and then stabilized before they can be transferred. It was a common practice for physician's to perform a "wallet biopsy" and determine that the patient could not pay and then transfer them to a tertiary center for care, regardless of their condition.

I highly suspected that the young man would die en-route, if he did not receive any blood. I finally succeeded in obtaining a central line, and the blood was given. We transferred the young man to Charlotte and he survived the episode. I suppose it was naïve, but I was appalled at the willingness of some people to let others die. Maybe I was wrong and he would have lived anyway— but why gamble on someone else's life.

There was another case that caused me a lot of concern. I was on duty in the ER, when some of the Intensive Care nurses showed me a patient's EKG (heart tracing). They had concerns about her rhythm and wanted my opinion. I told them that I thought she a second degree heart block and I was afraid that if anyone gave her lidocaine (a heart rhythm drug) for her PVC's (extra heart beats) that she would advance to a third degree block and die. It appeared to me that at this point she needed a pacemaker, which meant transfer.

Her local physician discovered that I had looked at the chart and the patient and had expressed an opinion for treatment—one that conflicted with his decisions. He met me in the ER and demanded that I stay out of the intensive care unit, away from his patients, and remain in the ER where I belonged. A few hours later, the lady had more PVC's and lidocaine was ordered. The woman went into third degree block and died.

I reviewed the chart the next day and found that the controversial EKG's were gone. I found that extremely interesting, but as I had been told, it was "not my case". Later in my career, I found this episode to be ironic, because in another case I was accused of altering medical records, which is a felony. So I chose not to say anything and nothing was done. It is an old saying that "a doctor buries his mistakes". I guess there is some truth to that.

On a lighter note, I was on duty once when a Code Blue (cardio-pulmonary arrest) presented to the ER. The on-call room was next door in the old Nurses Dormitory and as usual I got up and began to run to the emergency department. I had been relaxing—sleeping— between patients. I had learned to grab any sleep whenever you could, because it might have to last awhile. I discovered a slight problem. I was pretty young and disposed to those early morning erections that often occur in younger men. Well, I had a very obvious erection and the scrub pants only made it more obvious. I could not really delay responding, but the erection would not relax. When I arrived in the ER, the nurses just burst into laughter and pointed at my crotch. What are you going to do? I ran the code, the erection disappeared, and the patient lived.

Another case taught me to think twice before giving advice to patients on how they should live their lives. The patient was a beautiful young woman whom I had seen several times for various fractured (broken) bones. She came to the ER with another forearm fracture. I questioned her and it seemed that her husband was the responsible assailant. He would routinely get fairly drunk, drag her out of their trailer, beat her, throw her in the car and drive around town. I was astonished that she would tolerate that kind of behavior and suggested that she leave him, take the kids and go live with her mother. She cried that she was afraid of what he might do. I replied that she should not continue living in those circumstances.

After a few months, and another few incidents, she took my advice and went to her mother's. Apparently, the husband followed her, killed her and her mother, and took the kids. She had taken out all the correct legal warrants, restraining orders and followed the law, but that did not really help, she was still dead.

I left this ER and went back to Medical School, where I hoped to finish my residency in Internal Medicine. I ran out of money again, finished another year, and went back to work in the ER. It was 1983, and this time, I was lucky and got a position in the gorgeous Appalachian Mountains. I was so excited. This new ER was very busy and I was back to working 24 hour shifts, but I was in the mountains.

One of the local doctors had opened his practice just after World War II. He would tell me stories of "the old days" when he would make rounds in his aged car. Often, he was the only physician around. He talked about delivering babies at the patient's home. He would tell me that he often had to get a local sheriff to ride along because some of the places he had to go to were not very friendly to strangers. They ran into "moonshiners" on a regular basis. Many of the "hill" people were suspicious of strangers. I have always been fascinated with history, so it was great fun to hear his stories.

By the time I worked this next job, I had been practicing a few years and was starting to get a bit sure of myself. One night, a very large woman drove to the ER and developed cardiac arrest (her heart stopped) in the parking lot. One of the nurses and I ran out to the car and I began pulling her out. It is amazing how difficult it can be to stop "dead weight" once you get it moving. This unconscious woman was very heavy, and soon I was just trying to break her fall.

When I had her on the pavement, I began to perform mouth-to-mouth resuscitation. We no longer do this too much, but old habits are hard to break. I have a lot of trouble just watching a patient who has stopped breathing while everyone looks for an Ambu bag (a self-inflating bag with a face-mask for ventilations). The patient had apparently just eaten and she vomited a large amount of material into my mouth. I remember blowing food chunks out of my nose later.

I continued one-man CPR and the nurse came back with a wheeled stretcher. Next came the hard part. There were only three of us to lift this very large woman onto the stretcher. I got between her enormous thighs and the nurses each took a shoulder. We finally managed to get her on the stretcher and rolled her into the ER. We got an IV going, intubated her, and delivered some medicines. She responded well, came around, was extubated and admitted. She was able to return home fairly soon. Sometimes, not often, these things actually work well for the patient.

On another occasion, the ambulance brought in a gentleman with chest pain. He was pale, diaphoretic (sweating), and holding his chest. It was a classic myocardial infarction (heart attack) presentation. He had been experiencing the chest pain for about one hour. He was an out-of-town traveling salesman, in his mid-forties, and his girlfriend had come to visit him at the local hotel. They had been making love when the pain began.

It was such a wonderfully classic story and to top it all off, he was a very funny guy. He was in much pain and very scared, but he managed to tell me that "he always wanted to die in the saddle". We did all the usual medical maneuvers, but they did not work. He died. He had gotten his wish.

The girlfriend was crying and very emotional. She felt that it was all her fault. I assured her that she was not the cause of his heart disease and that it had all been a terrible coincidence. She began to feel a bit better.

Another episode reminded me to be reluctant to volunteer. A young woman with leukemia came into the ER from her local doctor's office. She had a severe anemia (low blood count) and he was going to transfer her for a transfusion. I spoke up and offered to start a central line (deep IV line) for the transfusion, hoping to make the transfer trip unnecessary. I had performed this procedure many times by now, with no complications, and really thought that I was helping.

To accomplish this procedure, one option is to use the deep vein in the neck- the internal carotid. I chose this method, prepped her in the usual manner, and stuck a very large needle in her neck. One known complication of this procedure is to miss the vein and hit the artery instead. I had never before hit the artery (and never did for the rest of my career) but this time I did puncture the artery. This is not usually a big problem. One can simply apply pressure to stop any bleeding and choose another site. This time, however, the artery kept bleeding and the resulting hematoma (collection of blood under the skin) continued to expand. I kept holding pressure.

The nurse, who was a friend of mine, and I looked at each other and asked aloud- "What now". I reviewed her lab work quickly and noticed the platelet count of 15,000. Platelets help a person clot their blood. This was a very low platelet count and I had made a huge mistake. I am not really sure why the local physician had failed to comment on the extremely low platelet count, but I learned to always review pertinent lab-work myself before attempting to help another physician. Thankfully, the bleeding stopped, the patient did fine, but she got transferred for any future therapeutic maneuvers.

Another lesson came from a young woman involved in a car wreck. This woman came in after she had been in an accident. Most of her injuries were simple cuts and scrapes, but she was very drunk. I remember that she kept rolling around on the ER bed and revealing her extremely distinct, flamboyant underwear. After I had examined her and ruled out any serious injury, I discharged her. I failed to go to the waiting room and determine how she had arrived at the ER. Her boyfriend, the driver, appeared to be extremely intoxicated, according to the nurses later that night.

There was a fatal car wreck later that night, and I was called to go obtain some blood from the victim. The police had been unable to identify the victim due to the horrendous extent of the injuries. As soon as I saw the underwear, I knew the victim's identity. I told the police. Another lesson learned. So what if I had been "busy"— I should have checked on her mode of transportation. Perhaps the nurse could have checked, or maybe the secretary. Sadly, it was too late for this woman. She was dead.

I had an incident that reminded me that just because a person had trained at an "elite" medical school, they were not necessarily good. I have always been impressed, and a little intimidated, by those who had the good fortune to attend a prestigious school. I had a patient in the ED, who had suffered a large heart attack. He was already demonstrating signs of heart failure. I knew that his only chance to live would require his transfer to a larger institution for care. I discussed the case with the on-call medical physician, who had trained at Duke. I expected to get the green light for a transfer. Instead, he suggested giving the man some nitroglycerin tablets sublingually (under the tongue) for his chest pain. In the doctor's defense, nitroglycerin is a drug that is often used in heart attack patients. I replied that perhaps he had not heard me state that the patient's blood pressure was already low. Nitroglycerin almost always makes the blood pressure drop. He said that he understood, but I needed to give him the nitroglycerin anyway, because "sometimes you have to sacrifice the heart, to save the patient".

I refused to administer any nitroglycerin and thought to myself, *did they teach you that at Duke?* The physician came to the ER, gave the patient some nitroglycerin. Then he spent the next hour trying to get his blood pressure back up to a level that was safe for transport. I did not hear any more about that case. I was no longer impressed with his "prestigious" education.

At this ER, the ambulances were staffed with basic EMT's (emergency medical technicians). These men and women took it on themselves to attend classes, learn new skills and upgrade to full paramedics. I was so proud of them, and the enormous dedication and sacrifice that they brought to the job. I assisted them and advocated for them as a medical supervisor for their training program. We had a large battle with the local county commissioners over their compensation, but we finally won. The commissioners had been happy to have their picture in the paper with the new "paramedics", but they wished to continue the pay at the old basic EMT level. We were not asking for the moon, but just the average salary for a paramedic in the state. These people had worked hard for their new status and they deserved the pay, in my opinion.

Along the same line, we needed new ambulances and some equipment, but we could not convince the commissioners. Things had gotten so bad, that when we transported someone to the larger hospital, we began to station a second ambulance about half-way along the route for the anticipated ambulance breakdown. I told the paramedics that we might get the equipment when one of the commissioners needed the service. This very thing finally happened and we did get the equipment. Sometimes you just have to wait for things to be right.

Another night and another shift, this time a deputy brought a prisoner in for an exam. The handcuffs had been removed for the exam, and I was almost finished, when the prisoner hit me and I fell back. He grabbed the deputy's gun, pushed him back, jumped over the front desk and took the secretary hostage. Another officer arrived and a gunfight ensued. The secretary and officers were not hurt, but the prisoner had been shot. Now, I had a gunshot wound to the chest to care for. We got him stabilized and called the local surgeon, who took him to the operating room for definitive treatment.

There was a lot of physical violence within this ER, and usually not a week went by without some sort of physical altercation. One evening, a very large "mountain" man had brought in his mother (his "Mama") down the mountain, to our facility. We had just gotten her situated in a bed, the chart assembled, and I was heading her way next, when he became belligerent. He was drunk, and he loudly began to harass some of the ER nurses about Mama.

I was not about to let him hurt one of the nurses, so I stepped in and tried to address his concerns. He thought we were taking too long to see his mother. I calmly explained that his mother had just gotten back, and was the next patient to be seen. This explanation did not help, and he lunged at me. He swung a fist and I ducked. He missed and our secretary grabbed me and hustled me off "to see another patient". She had intervened to save me from being badly beaten. About this time, his mother yelled out "Robert, you leave that doctor alone and let them go about their business".

"Yes, mama" was all he could say, as he tried to find a seat. Thank God, for maternal guidance!

There was a recurring problem in the ER that I needed to resolve: overcrowding of the treatment area with concerned family and friends. Often, after an accident victim arrived in the ER, the family and friends would appear and pack into the trauma room. While I understood their concern, their presence made it impossible to properly assess and care for the victim. I understood that they all wanted to see the victim and let them know that they were there for them. However, the victim was often in critical condition and I really needed access to establish the extent of injuries, and treat any immediately life-threatening conditions that might be present. I would resolve this issue by making an announcement to the crowd that "I will come in, when all of you are finished visiting". Most of the time, this announcement was enough to encourage members of the crowd to assist in clearing the room. Soon, they would invite me to "come on in".

As I said earlier, this was a rural mountain community and some of the patients were definitely different from what I was comfortable with. There were a couple of families that were well-known to the ER staff. These families made a lot of moonshine liquor and engaged in a lot of inbreeding. Once, the grandfather brought his granddaughter in for some ailment. I examined her and could not help noticing that she was very pregnant. She was only about 14 years old, and this was her second pregnancy. The grandfather was the father of the child. I could not restrain myself from asking him why he would do this to his own grand-daughter. He never really answered my question and the behavior did not change. All of the appropriate agencies already knew this family well, but the behavior persisted.

Another patient introduced me to the phrase *stump-jumping,* which I was unfamiliar with. This man would arrive in the ER two or three times a year with bird-shot in his back from a shot-gun blast. The injuries were not serious. It turns out that stump-jumping was a man committing bestiality with a cow. The perpetrator would back a cow up to a tree stump and then climb onto the stump to perform the act. The farmer who owned the cow would sometimes catch him in the "act", yell at him to get off the cow, and then shoot him in the back with his shotgun as he fled the field. I suppose it takes all kinds, but that seems a little too strange.

I had another case that caused me a lot of anguish. A gentleman came to the ER with abdominal pain. He was in his mid-fifties and had a history of hypertension (high blood pressure). He was in obvious acute distress, pale and diaphoretic (sweating). When he first arrived, he was able to maintain a decent blood pressure, but that changed during the diagnostic work-up. Indeed, I was able to prove that he had a leaking abdominal aortic aneurysm (AAA). This is a very serious diagnosis and carries a very high mortality (death) rate with it.

I called the referral hospital ER and spoke with the receiving physician. As it happened, he was an old friend of mine. I told him about the patient and the diagnosis.

I requested a medical helicopter for transport. The phone was silent for a moment. Then my friend responded "Dr. Bentley, you know that he is going to die, right?" I said that of course I knew, but that he was still alive now— I could not just put him in the corner and let him die. He sent the helicopter and the man died while we were loading him. At least we had tried.

One Christmas, I was dispatched to another mountain town to cover its emergency department. It was extremely cold that day. The heater in my car did not work, so the drinking water I had with me froze. I arrived at the little town and checked into a local motel for the night. The motel owner was having problems also and his motel heat stopped running that night. In the morning, I got ready for the shift, but my car would not crank. The motel owner was already up trying to fix the heat, so he gave me a ride to the local hospital. He also agreed to pick me up the next morning. What a way to start a shift!

I met the staff and worked the shift. When things quieted down at about two in the morning, I found the on-call room and lay down for a break. After an hour or so, I was paged to the ER for a Code Blue (cardiac arrest). I ran out to the ER, but it was empty. I could not find anyone.

Then, I heard someone call out that the patient was out in the back, at the ER loading ramp. I ran outside, the temperature was in the teens, and I had mere scrubs on. I was standing there, trying to stay warm, and let my eyes adjust to the dim light. One of the nurses updated me. Apparently, a man—a patient— had been in the hospital and decided to leave. He had gotten into his truck, in the back parking lot, and started to drive away. Unfortunately for him, he had a heart attack, slumped over the steering wheel, and drove down a small hill into a tree. He had no pulse and no respirations, and they only found him because the horn was blaring.

Some of the staff were trying to assist him. They were trying to perform CPR, but I could see that he was still sitting up and no one was breathing for him. The chest percussions were being performed sideways, so of course, they were completely ineffectual. They finally got him out of the truck and onto a stretcher. As they tried to roll him up the hill, they continued CPR, but again no one was assisting his ventilations. They tried valiantly to roll him up the hill to the ER, but the body kept falling off the stretcher. They would then stop, in the dark and cold, pick up the limp figure, put it back on the stretcher, and set off for the ER again.

This happened several times. It truly resembled an episode of *Keystone Cops*. If it had not been so grave, it would have been hilarious. When they finally got to the ER, the patient was obviously dead, but my new ER associates were so solemn and had worked so hard that I started an IV, intubated the patient, and initiated a code. After a few minutes, I pronounced him dead and congratulated everyone on their monumental, but futile, effort.

Later, that same day, I was called to consult on a patient who was already in the hospital and being treated for pneumonia by her local physician. The woman was in her mid-fifties and was becoming more short of breath. I was called to examine her. I checked her vital signs (temperature, blood pressure, pulse and respirations – we did not have pulse oximetry then), examined her, read the chart and reviewed her chest x-ray. I concluded that she was suffering from congestive heart failure— not pneumonia, which, to my amazement, is what she was being treated for. The therapy for the two conditions is very different.

I began aggressively treating her congestive heart failure, and in about an hour or so, she could breathe much better. She thanked me. I spoke with her local doctor over the phone, and could not help being sarcastic. I explained what I had found, what I had done, and how perhaps, if he had been treating the right diagnosis, she might have been better this Christmas. He may have been a perfectly good doctor, but he did not know me, whether I was any good or not, and I was mad that he had not even come in to see his own patient.

On another occasion, when I had returned to my "home" hospital, it was late in the shift when the ambulance siren screamed in the night, and the radio announced that the paramedics were bringing in a young male victim from an auto accident. It seems that the young man was intoxicated and had driven off a bridge into a shallow river. He was not submerged, but actually, the cold water probably helped the man, because cold temperatures will decrease a person's metabolism and reduce the extent of any brain injuries. This young man had a small chunk of the bridge lodged deep in the left side of his head. It turns out that the head injury was his biggest problem. He was paralyzed, intubated and stabilized. All actively bleeding sites were repaired or bandaged, fractures were splinted, and he received the usual IV (intravenous) fluids to assist his blood pressure.

I talked with the physician at the receiving hospital and transferred the patient. It looked like things had gone pretty well, considering the extent of the head injury. I assumed he would die, but perhaps they could harvest some of the organs for donation.

Miraculously, he did not die. He survived, albeit with extensive neurological damage. He experienced rehab (rehabilitation) and was discharged home after a few months. I saw him again in the ER, as a patient, several times over the next two years. He was not at all grateful that he had survived. He was, in fact, very depressed and angry. He had become an enormous care burden for his parents and each time I saw him in the ER now, he had been trying, unsuccessfully, to commit suicide. I did not know the young man very well, but I could not help sympathizing about his condition. Yes, he had brought it on himself, but I still felt sorry for him. I might want to ask myself now: if I had known how it would turn out, would I have worked on him so hard when he first arrived? As an ER physician, however, that decision is not really mine to make, is it?

I had a similar experience later, when an older gentleman was shot at a local gun show. He came in by ambulance and we worked on him for a long while before we lost the battle and he died. Then, I found out "the rest of the story" as radio commentator Paul Harvey used to say. It seems that this man was shot, while running back to his truck to get his gun and shoot someone. I am glad that many times I don't know the whole story. It might influence my performance.

There was another incident that really stands out for me. Late one evening, a mother brought in her four adult sons. She was trying to have them committed to a mental institution. An ER doctor may commit a patient to a mental hospital if he determines that the patient is a danger to themselves or to others. As I told you earlier, moonshine stills were common in these parts.

It seems that the men had a still in the woods. They would run the still, drink some, and then sell the rest. Their mother disapproved of this behavior and had warned the "boys" that if they continued she would "have them all committed". Now the men were all pretty drunk. They laughed and giggled about their predicament. They kept slapping each other and giggling that "Ma is going to have us committed". The men were all in their thirties and their mom was in her early sixties. The mother kept trying to control her "boys", while threatening to "commit" during the entire visit.

There was no real physical problem with the men. I tried to explain to the mother that it was not against the law to drink in the woods. Besides, I was not the law and had no power to arrest them. I certainly wasn't going to commit them. The "boys" just laughed louder, and mom was furious. She really wanted to do something, but did not wish to get the "boys" in trouble with the law. I talked to the men, exhorting them to do the right thing, then I discharged them to return home with their mother.

I saw another case that was baffling. A woman in her mid-fifties came into the ER with atypical chest pain. Her vital signs were all normal and the physical was unrevealing. I had just read the EKG— it was normal. I was discussing the findings with her, as well as possible treatment options. As I watched,her eyes rolled back in her head and she "arrested" (cardiac arrest). I began CPR, intubated her, got an IV, and began to give some IV meds.

The on-call doctor, who was a friend of mine and had been the chief resident at Massachusetts General Hospital, came in to assist. Mass General is a prestigious hospital in medical circles. At first, he doubted that anyone with a "normal" EKG could arrest, but after reviewing the cardiogram he agreed. *Oh well*, I thought, *you live, and hopefully you learn.*

We succeeded in getting her back and he admitted her to the hospital. She did well, and eventually went home. Thrombolytic therapy (using clot-dissolving drugs) was still a few years in the future and not well thought of by many of the local doctors. In those days, the mid-1980's, the medical options for heart attack were very limited. Sometimes, things do change for the better.

I had another case that provided me with a "learning" experience. One night a young man lost control of his car and went off the side of the mountain. It was a convertible sports car and he had the top down. He was thrown from the auto as it rolled down the mountain. It was extremely difficult terrain for the EMS crew, but at last they got to him, brought him up to the ambulance, and hauled him to the ER.

On arrival he was in obvious extremis (dying). We quickly secured the airway and began several IV lines. Transfusion of blood was begun, due to the unresponsive hypotension (low blood pressure). His fractures had all been stabilized and all obvious bleeding had been controlled. I noticed, however, that blood was pooling up on the floor beneath him as fast as I was pouring it in. It was then that I corrected my error and rolled him up to examine the back. The skin and muscles had all been "filleted" off of most of his back, leaving the spine and ribs exposed. Obviously, this was the site of the massive bleeding. There was nothing else to do— the injuries were much too extensive. He was pronounced dead.

His parents ran a small restaurant that I used to pass on my drive home. I always thought of their son and felt sorry for their loss. Trauma courses, of course, teach one to examine the entire body, but I had not had one yet. This is one of the many problems that existed in the ER in the "early" days. Physicians of many different backgrounds were working emergency departments with no real emergency skills. A patient might see a dermatologist or endocrinologist. There were no real standards yet, but it was changing, and in my opinion, it was getting better. At least, it was getting better for the patients.

One of the pioneers of the Emergency Medicine specialty was Greg Henry, M.D. I was fortunate enough to have him for my oral boards later. Oral boards are a style of testing, where the applicant is given an emergency medicine scenario, and then has a specified time in which to assess and plan their approach to the problem. It can be a very anxiety-producing event. I had seen Dr. Henry before at numerous medical education courses and knew him to be intelligent, well-read, and quick-witted. He was respected as a leader in the new specialty of Emergency Medicine. His reputation was very intimidating and I suppose that like a lot of people, I was afraid that I would not measure up. I did fine.

The setting for the Oral Boards that year always seemed a bit odd to me. The boards were given at a hotel at O'Hare International airport. It was on the 6th floor. There was an open balcony at the end. There were all these ED doctor candidates, very scared and depressed, staring off this balcony. It seemed like a comical invitation for suicide. Fortunately, no one jumped.

It was another shift in the ER. It was very cold that night with temperatures in the teens. We had a freezing rain and the roads had become incredibly slick. The ambulances were having a difficult time of it. Often, on a slight incline on the roads, they would simply slide off into the ditch. It would seem like the perfect night to stay home and read or watch TV, but that was not to be. People got on the phone and called 911 all night, much of it for routine, minor physical complaints—which certainly could have waited until the roads were in better condition. They often had cars, but the weather was "too bad to get out" so they called an ambulance. There was a lot of action that night. People shot each other, stabbed each other, hit each other in the head with frying pans and a variety of other activities. I would not have guessed it.

It was late at night, on my last shift at this facility, when a car sped up to the ER unloading area. They dumped out a body, screamed that he had been shot, and then raced off into the night. The patient was a young man with multiple bullet wounds in his chest and abdomen. We loaded him onto a stretcher and wheeled him into the trauma room in the emergency department. A quick survey revealed that he was unconscious, still breathing, but already in hypovolemic shock (low blood volume, low blood pressure, and high pulse rate). We rapidly intubated him, placed bilateral (both sides) chest tubes, and inserted a variety of peripheral and central (deep veins) IV lines for volume replacement. We began transfusing him as soon as the laboratory could get the blood. Despite all our good efforts, the young man expired. Well, all you can do is try.

I really enjoyed working in a small-town emergency department, but my educational debts were not getting any smaller and I was rapidly heading toward my 40's. I had been paying on my school debts since I was 25, but it was obvious that I needed to make a change in my life. So I decided to take a high-paying big city job, and I left the mountains.

CHAPTER 6

ER Medicine in the Big City

MY NEW JOB WAS ACTUALLY A huge improvement for me. Within a few years my medical school debts were paid and I finally began to work for me. I was not used to the educated patients taking an interest in their health problems, but I quickly learned to like it.

This emergency department had plenty of equipment to work with. That was a pleasant change. Many of the older ER's lacked equipment such as patient heart monitors, digital blood pressure machines, pulse oximeters (to show oxygen level in the blood). They often lacked even basic orthopedic equipment such as rapidly adjustable crutches, Velcro splints, or walking ankle splints. Modern and more equipment improved the job conditions, but it was still stressful ER medicine.

This was in the mid-1980's, and the AID's epidemic was gaining momentum. I saw many patients with their first "opportunistic" infection (infections that afflict people with suppressed immune systems). Usually, this was pneumonia from the *Pneumocystis* organism. At that time, the HIV diagnosis was a death sentence. We were extremely vigilant about incurring needle stick injuries with possible blood exposure. I don't recall anyone refusing to care for a patient because of HIV, but there were a lot of unknowns. The ER staff were appropriately cautious when it came to bodily fluids.

On one shift, I had a patient who required a subclavian IV (in the deep central vein). To accomplish this procedure, the operator has to stick the large vein, thread a guide-wire down, remove the needle, then thread the indwelling IV catheter into the vein. Rarely, have I ever stuck myself while performing this procedure, but this time I did. The patient was an ex-convict with multiple tattoos. I was working myself into a real panic as I stared at the blood on the needle and at the patient. I thought, *why couldn't you be a little nun from one of the nursing homes*? The patient saw my anxious appearance and said "it is OK Doc. I just got tested for AIDS last week and it was negative".

Thank God!

Every ED doctor has a —foreign body in the rectum— story. I have one that stands out for me. Actually, this diagnosis is much too common. I have been thinking of getting a law passed that would require manufacturers of commonly used rectal objects, to place a ring on the end of the object, to assist in the removal of the object from the rectum. This is the story of an older gentleman, who strikingly resembled Santa Claus. It was just before Christmas. That fact made it even worse for me. He was married, but that night he was with his girlfriend. Apparently, his wife did not enjoy the use of sex toys. I had a disturbing picture of "Grandma" sitting at home alone, in her rocking chair.

Anyway, he had this long, wooden dildo lodged in his rectum. I would have thought that splinters would be an issue. The object had slipped from his hand. Lord, I worked for several hours to get that dildo. It was very slippery, and the colon holds it back with a vacuum-like suction. If I was unable to remove it in the ED, then he would have to undergo surgery. I am not judgmental, but it all seemed so wrong. I had my hand up "Santa's" ass, trying to fish out a wooden dildo. Grandma was at home; and Christmas was approaching fast. *I suppose it takes all kinds.*

I finally succeeded in retrieving the object and I was about to throw it away, when he asked if he could have it back. "Why not", I simply replied.

Early one evening, during a shift, a teenage girl was brought into the ER by ambulance. Her vital signs (blood pressure, pulse, respiratory rate) were all normal, but she had a fever. She was delirious, talking out of her head and it was not clear what was causing her symptoms. A quick history from the mother effectively excluded recent head injury or drug abuse, but just to be sure, the proper tests were ordered. You know the old saying from Ronald Reagan about diplomacy with the Soviets – "Trust, but verify." Apparently, the girl had seen her local doctor earlier that day for "cold-like" symptoms and he had been unimpressed. I ordered a battery of blood tests and prepped her for a spinal tap— it was definitely indicated.

A spinal tap sounds a bit frightening. It is really just gathering another bodily fluid for evaluation. Yes, the needle goes in the back. It is pretty far down from the end of the spinal cord, so there is almost no chance of paralysis. A local anesthetic is injected first, so the pain that is associated with a spinal tap is usually minimal.

In this case, the tap was impressive. The cerebrospinal fluid is usually clear, like water from a faucet, but this fluid was very cloudy and viscous. Indeed, she had severe bacterial meningitis and I immediately started intravenous broad-spectrum antibiotics as well as steroids for the inflammation. Usually, with symptoms this severe, and overwhelming infection, the patient will have neurologic sequelae (residual neurologic symptoms), if they manage to survive the episode. I am happy to report that this young girl did very well. She survived and there were no detectable neurologic deficits. Her doctor had not missed anything. He just saw her early in her disease process.

Over the next few weeks, several of her classmates came by the ER to thank me. It turns out that she was some sort of local soccer star. I was just thankful that she made it, but it was gratifying to see the outpouring of emotion from her classmates.

I had another case that had a tragic ending. A young man (early twenties) came in with flu-like symptoms. There was nothing out of the ordinary in his symptoms and the physical exam was completely normal, but my sub-conscious alarms were buzzing. So I ordered a lot of tests, often referred to as a "fishing expedition". Everything came back negative— blood tests, chest ray, urine—but the alarms continued to ring.

I finally performed a spinal tap to look at the spinal fluid, even though he really did not have any physical indications for this exam. I wanted to be completely thorough. All the tests were negative—they said only that he was a healthy young male. I reflected that perhaps I was wrong after all. I discharged him with a diagnosis of "viral illness."

A few hours later, he rolled back in by ambulance. This time he was dead. He had died at home. I was incredulous. *How had this happened? Everything was completely normal.*

I learned then, what a virulent organism *Neisseria meningitides* really could be. According to the autopsy reports, apparently the infection had been so widespread, and rapid, that his body never had the time necessary to mount a defense. So there was no elevated white count, no pneumonia— not even the expected meningitis. It just over-ran the individual, and killed him. It was truly an amazing organism.

A local newspaper columnist got the story and printed an article that implied that the boy had come to the ER, nothing was done, and he was sent home to die. I was furious. The columnist had not even mentioned that the boy had undergone extensive evaluation and testing, including a spinal tap, before he was discharged. It is impossible to admit everyone with only a low-grade fever.

I was so angry with the story that I called and talked to her. I commented that I had read the article, but that it had failed to tell the entire story. I related the other facts of what had happened. She admitted that she had not interviewed anyone from the ER before releasing the story. All of my peers— doctor friends— commented that I should "just let it go" and that I was only going to make the situation worse, but I disagreed. I thought that the truth did matter. The next week, the columnist printed a fuller account of the events, exonerating me and the hospital and discussing how devastating an infection Neisseria can be. Sometimes, the truth hurts, but it is still the truth.

I found the next case to be incredibly disturbing. A woman in her early twenties was at home, when a man, who had been stalking her, burst through the kitchen door, grabbed a knife, chased her down, and stabbed her multiple times in both sides of her chest. She came in by ambulance. Her vital signs were good, except for a tachycardia (fast heart rate). The breath sounds were equal on both sides of the chest, which suggested that the lungs were still inflated and not perforated (pneumothorax).

The information that I received was that the man had seen the woman's picture in a high school yearbook and began stalking her.

The chest x-ray was normal, so it appeared that the knife had not penetrated her skin and fatty tissue deeply enough to and cut into the lungs or heart. She was very large breasted: perhaps this anatomy had served as a buffer to stop the knife from penetrating further, I thought. My feelings of concern about her began to ease somewhat, since it appeared that there were just multiple small skin lacerations to repair.

The girl began to look very frightened, which was to be expected after all she had been through. But she began to complain that she could not breathe. I quickly looked at the chest x-ray again. It was normal. I assured her that it was just a sensation, that everything looked fine. She looked up at me, cried out, and then arrested (her heart and lungs stopped). I quickly swung into action, but my mind was frantically racing—what had I missed?

I began CPR and set-up for bilateral chest tubes. Once I made the incision in her side and the first chest tube went in, a large amount of blood came pouring out. There was so much blood, that at first I thought somehow I had stuck the tube in her heart, but that was not the answer. I raced to the other side of the chest, stuck in a tube, and out poured more blood. Where was all this blood coming from? The chest x-ray had been negative. We began immediate blood transfusions. Repeat CXR showed good chest tube placement, and both lungs were inflated. The patient began to respond, but she could not speak, because by now she was intubated. Her blood pressure was coming up and that was great.

We called the on-call surgeon to take her to the OR and open her chest. He arrived and said"good job". I saw him later, after the surgery, and asked about the injuries.

Apparently, the knife had entered from the side of the chest, passed through the lungs, and struck the heart several times, resulting in multiple stab wounds to her heart. I always try to review each big case of mine, trying to learn for the next case. It did not seem feasible that a well-taken x-ray would have failed to disclose her extensive internal injuries. I learned that if the CXR (chest x-ray) is obtained in a semi-erect position (partially sitting up) too soon after the injury, the blood may be hidden, but still collecting. I still don't understand how the lungs could sustain multiple stab wounds and remain inflated—that is not supposed to happen.

The woman survived the assault for a few more days, but then she died from her injuries.

I was summoned to her murder trial, where I saw the murder weapon for the first time. I began to better understand the pathophysiology of her injuries. The murder weapon was a very long, thin knife. The killer had apparently stabbed her in both sides of her chest. The knife penetrated her lungs and entered the heart. It was a long distance, but it was a very long knife. When I first saw her, it had seemed that her large breasts had saved her, and with a regular knife, they might have done just that.

Another case I encountered was very sad. This case was also extremely bewildering to me. Late one night, the ambulance brought in a young, healthy looking male. His initial history was consistent with another routine viral illness or cold. It was that time of year, so it was to be expected. As I said, his vital signs were fine, except for a mild fever (101), and he was alert and joking.

Suddenly, he began to feel faint. His BP had dropped. He was becoming more and more lethargic (comatose). I moved rapidly, trying to consider all the possible explanations and then some. There had been no head injury, so I could essentially rule that out as a cause. He became comatose and required intubation and ventilation. This was accomplished, but I was still searching for the etiology (cause). He was young, in his early thirties, and had no significant past medical history. The spinal tap was negative, as were all the x-ray's and head CT, but he was dying. I continued to ask, *What is going on?*

His wife was a beautiful young woman, and they had recently gotten married. Their whole future together was just beginning. There were holidays, family, kids, traveling and generally living. She was frantic and kept looking to me for help. I was trying. His BP began to crash and we started a dopamine drip (intravenous medicine to elevate the BP).

Feverishly, I continued to wrack my brain for a possible etiology— something, anything, that would explain all of this. But I could not think of anything. We lost the race and he died. His wife was sobbing. It was all over, and I still did not know what had happened.

The young widow was extremely distraught. She asked if she could clip a lock of his hair to keep. "Of course", I replied," he is your husband".

His body was sent for an autopsy. The pathologist and I knew each other well. He said "Dr. Bentley, you could not have saved him, even if you had known what was happening, it was too late. He had Coxsackie viral myocarditis, and had bled all through is heart. Sorry."

Jesus, I thought. I had never even heard of it before, so I began reading. Usually, the Coxsackie virus causes a mild "viral" illness, like a cold, and the patient recovers. Rarely, it can infect the heart muscle and result in myocarditis (heart infection) with diffuse hemorrhaging and heart failure. Again, I was extremely impressed with the microbial world. I had given the man's widow my home phone number because I felt so bad for her. She called several times, over the next few months, usually crying and begging me to explain to her what had happened. I initially gave her the technical explanation, and eventually just explained that he was "unlucky". I am sure you have heard the expression that life is not fair, but sometimes it just sucks.

I was in my mid-forties now, and the year was 1994. I received the chance to experience my second malpractice lawsuit. This time it involved a patient that I had never even seen face to face; in fact, he had not come through the emergency department. The patient had been in the hospital under the care of one of the local doctors, when the patient developed increasing abdominal pain. The local doctor kept treating him, over the phone, with pain medicine, but he was getting worse. All the nurses and the ancillary staff could tell, walking by the room, that he was very ill.

Finally, the local doctor consulted a general surgeon, again over the phone. The general surgeon ordered an abdominal x-ray over the phone and went back to bed. He did not come in either.

Before the surgeon went back to bed, he called me in the ED and asked if I would look at the x-ray as a favor. I did not know the patient; I had never seen the patient. But I knew the surgeon and agreed to look at the x-ray as a courtesy. After I reviewed the x-ray, I called the surgeon at home, and said "The x-ray looks really bad. I think he has a small bowel obstruction (blocked bowel) with dilated loops of bowel". I continued "I think you need to see this guy".

The surgeon chose to continue treating the patient with intra-muscular pain meds, and went back to bed. Unfortunately for the patient, he perforated (ruptured) his bowel and died. The prosecuting lawyers found my name in the chart where I had read the x-ray for the surgeon and included me in the lawsuit.

On my initial visit, I explained to the lawyers that I had never even seen the patient, but I spent the next three years hiring my own lawyers and preparing my defense. Finally, one of the lawyers looked up from his sheet of paper and said "You never even saw the patient". I agreed with him, and pointed out that I had told them that three years before. Subsequently, I was dismissed from the lawsuit. Apparently, the lawsuit had been on "autopilot" for three years, and finally, after someone reviewed the case, I had been dismissed. What a system!

Some patients have a disease that is difficult to diagnose. But there are some patients for whom it is impossible to diagnose a disease—because they don't have one. Patients present with faked illnesses all the time. It really makes the job much harder when, as a doctor, you must determine whether the symptoms are real. Quite often, we physicians, never comprehend the secondary gain that a particular patient is seeking. The secondary gain can range from drug seeking, attention seeking, or some other goal such as avoiding court. This is one of the reasons that pediatric practice is so appealing; most children are too young to fake a serious illness, other than to avoid school, and that particular subterfuge is usually obvious and easy to determine.

Take, for example the pretended seizure in an adult. When the physician is inexperienced, and the patient is an expert at faking, it can be difficult to differentiate the real from the not-real. I had one patient who would stop his seizure long enough to sign the registration forms, and then resume seizing. Obviously, this type of voluntary control is impossible in a real seizure. As the physician acquires more years of experience, it becomes easier to distinguish a true seizure from a simulated one.

Another favorite diagnosis for patients to try and mimic is paralysis. This diagnosis can be very difficult to deal with, and when there is an experienced and uncooperative faker, this encounter can result in a lot of unnecessary testing. It is difficult, if not impossible, to prove a negative. If the patient says they can't move their legs, then unless you are able to trick them into moving, you must assume that the patient is telling the truth.

One patient of mine with "paralyzed legs" comes to mind. She rolled into the ER, by ambulance, with her legs held high in the air, screaming to everyone that she was paralyzed. She was not, of course, but it is often difficult to convince the patient that you know he or she is not paralyzed. In this case, I remembered her from the week before, during another visit. I informed her that her gonorrhea culture had been positive. Upon hearing this news, she jumped off the stretcher, cursed her "boyfriend" and ran out of the ER threatening to "kill that SOB". Another paralysis case was cured. She followed up the gonorrhea diagnosis at a later date.

Emergency staff often must also determine if a patient is feigning unconsciousness. One case of mine, in this category, inspired real admiration. She was very good. A young woman, in her mid-thirties, had boarded a Greyhound Bus in New York City and traveled down I-95 to my town, where she suddenly became comatose (unconscious) and paralyzed, according to witnesses. She was brought into my ER, by ambulance, and I began to search for etiologies. She had the "fluttering eye" sign (eyelids twitching when someone purposely keeps their eyes shut). This usually indicates a feigned coma, but we could not get her to awaken or move.

There are a variety of methods that a doctor or nurse can perform that usually provoke a response in an uncooperative patient who is really awake. An ammonia capsule in the nostril is one, but if the patient is experienced, they will simply breathe out of their mouth and avoid the ammonia. I anticipated this and held my hand over her mouth, thus forcing her to breathe through her nose. She had tears streaming out of those fluttering eyes, but she would not open her eyes or move.

I had already run the necessary coma tests and they were all negative. I was sure she was faking, but I could not prove it without her cooperation. I finally gave up and called the admitting physician, presented the case, and had her admitted.

A few days later, she still was not responding, and the local physician was aggravated. He discharged her, poured her into a wheelchair and rolled her out if front of the hospital. After an hour or so, when she still would not respond, he went out, brought her back in and readmitted her. He did not know what else to do.

Two days later, the patient "woke" up and left the hospital AMA (against medical advice). She was last seen running to the bus station, with her hospital gown open in the back and blowing in the breeze. It turns out that she had been avoiding a court date in Columbia, S.C. She now had a valid medical excuse. I have seen a lot of fakes in my career, but she was truly impressive.

A few years ago, the JCAH (joint commission on accreditation of hospitals) released a statement that said, in so many words, that there are no drug seeking patients in the emergency department, but only undertreated patients. I don't know where they have been practicing, but in my emergency departments, there have been many drug seeking patients. The person may be an addict or someone involved in drug dealing—or both. Often, the nurses will comment that a particular patient is "just here for drugs". As a doctor, one must always understand that even these patients can be sick. However, most of the long-time nurses are very familiar with their patient population. Personally, I try not to prejudge any patient seeking emergency services. I have always taken the approach that I would rather pass out a few undeserved narcotic prescriptions, than to miss one real patient who needs my help.

There are a couple of diagnoses that have become favorites of the drug-seeking crowd. These are headaches and back pain, for a simple reason: it is impossible to know if the complaint is real or simply an attempt to obtain narcotic prescriptions. I am not a judgmental person. I am a child of the Sixties, so I am tolerant of people who choose to take drugs. But I say *Let them buy them on the street like we did and avoid the enormous medical costs to society.* It is not uncommon to see the same individual 2 or 3 times in a day, by ambulance, complaining of pain. Then, they take a few prescribed pills for themselves and sell the rest on the street. These individuals are always allergic to all other drugs, except the one drug that they prefer.

Finally, I will address one other issue regarding patient misuse of emergency medical resources. Most counties only have 3 or 4 ambulances. On busy days or nights, accident victims and others with acute medical emergencies, must wait longer while the ambulance crews respond to earlier requests for assistance. When these delays are caused by patients without true emergencies, people may die. I think that this is wrong. Many, but not all, counties now have a policy that the paramedics can decide whether to transport or not. If there is any doubt at all, then simply transport. But if they have already been to a particular residence several times that day, and they know that the patient is stable, then they may refuse to transport. After all, paramedics are trained medical personnel and are accustomed to making medical decisions.

CHAPTER 7

Back to Small-town ER Medicine

WHEN I WAS IN MY LATE forties, I decided to return to my emergency department roots. I took a job in a small town, rural hospital ER. It was like stepping back in time. The department had little equipment, and what it had was pretty outdated. It was a challenge. There was minimal staff and in this facility, and the doctor had to leave the ED to go hunt down an x-ray. This practice is a cardinal sin in more modern facilities. Ideally, an emergency physician is expected to be persistently available for any need or crisis of ER patients, and that is not possible if the physician is in another part of the hospital. Another sign of the backwardness in this ED was that they still used the old wooden crutches. These required about thirty minutes of assembly time. I found myself, assembling crutches, and pondering that the hospital was paying a board-certified physician to assemble crutches. I was glad to do it for the benefit of the patients, but it seemed like a big waste of finances.

Inefficient practices at this hospital sometimes put the ER patients at risk. One time, a critical patient with a gunshot wound to the chest waited for an x-ray, while the x-ray technician pursued her schedule of previously ordered x-ray's for the in-house patients. I had to exit the ED, find the x-ray technician, and tell her to come to the ED immediately for my emergency patient. She protested the interruption, but came to the ED at my strong suggestion.

Still, it was interesting to be back in a small-town rural ED, because there is always such a wide variety of pathology to deal with. Eventually, with a lot of constructive criticism from me about our equipment, the facility began to acquire equipment that was more modern.

I think that I am particularly evolved for work in the emergency department. As I mentioned, the disease that I have, Kartagener's Syndrome, includes chronic sinusitis and chronic bronchitis. What this means practically for my work in the ER, is that I can't smell anything. Thus, I am great for "digging out" fecal impactions (stool backed up in the rectum) and draining anaerobic abscesses (infections without oxygen). Apparently, these particular diagnoses have a very bad odor associated with them, but they don't bother me. The nurses are always eager to have me "dig out" the fecal impactions, because this is a particularly unpleasant chore. By the way, it is very uncomfortable for the patients too.

I was draining a large pilonidal cyst (abscess in the fold of the buttocks) one day, and assisted by one of the ER nurses. With my back to the nurse, I requested some additional sponges for all the pus draining out. There was no response. I asked for the sponges again, but nothing happened. I turned to look and realized that I was alone in the room with the patient. I found the nurse outside at the desk. She said that the odor was overwhelming and that she was about to pass out. I told her it was alright and I finished draining the abscess by myself. Oh well, at least she tried to help.

One morning, I was driving down the Interstate, on my way to work. I glanced at a young man on the side of the road who was staggering and appeared drunk. Shortly after I arrived in the ED, the ambulance announced that they were bringing the young man into the ED because of a stab wound. After a quick, initial exam, it appeared that the stab wound over the anterior (front) left chest, was the only injury. His vital signs were stable. He was breathing on his own, and the lungs sounded by auscultation (listening with a stethoscope) as if they were both inflated.

The man smelled and acted very drunk and was unable to provide any helpful history. I continued to listen to his chest and was sure that I could hear a Hamann's Crunch (a crunching sound that occurs with the heartbeat indicating air around the heart). I reviewed the CXR hard, but could not see any evidence of air in the pericardium (sack around the heart). The man remained stable.

We transferred him to another facility, Duke, for further imaging studies. The receiving trauma surgeon at Duke Hospital was cordial when I talked with him on the phone, but admitted that he was not familiar with a Hamann's Crunch. It is an old term that is taught in most trauma courses, but perhaps by that time it had become outdated.

I explained the significance of the term and he accepted the patient. The patient did well and further testing was negative. Perhaps, I was just hearing things. Better safe than sorry.

Another shift began on a rocky note. As I was driving into the hospital, I got behind a bus loaded with Hispanics. The bus turned toward the hospital and continued down the road. It got closer to the hospital, and finally turned into the ER parking lot. I could not help thinking, *Oh, this is just great! A busload of non-English speaking Hispanics to start my day.* I am happy to treat all races and nationalities. But I spoke only *poquito* (a little) Spanish. This was a small-town ER and we certainly did not have interpreters.

It turned out that only one of the passengers needed medical help. This gentleman was a heroin addict. The bus had left Mexico a day earlier, and he had run out of heroin. Now, he was in acute withdrawal. Heroin withdrawal is not usually fatal, but it is very unpleasant. I took care of the young man, he got back on the bus and it continued on to New York City.

I have always been impressed with people who can't understand the doctor (me), but will allow me to do very complex and sometimes painful procedures to them. Dealing with persons who speak only languages other than English has become a large problem in the ED. Most small-town hospitals cannot afford to provide a full-time interpreter. In addition to those who speak Spanish, there may be those who speak other languages such as Mandarin, Japanese, French, Russian and many others. By definition, many emergency room patients have experienced some traumatic event, and an added challenge for some is the enormous language barrier when they request medical help.

I remember one Hispanic patient who had been brought in by ambulance and needed a chest tube placed. I had no time to wait for an interpreter to be found or called. He spoke no English. I could only speak a little Spanish. With my limited Spanish I tried to tell him what I needed to do. All I could come up with was to say *"grande dolor"* (big pain) and gesture for him to try to hold still. He stayed motionless and let me perform the procedure. If the tables were reversed, I don't think that I would allow a stranger, who I could not understand, pierce my chest and insert a big plastic tube. I believe that people who want to make their home in America should speak English, but the reality is that some do not. We doctors should still take care of them.

There was another incident that just broke my heart. A woman in her mid-forties was coming home from a kayaking vacation in western North Carolina. She was married with a few children. They were traveling on an interstate highway, outside of town, when they passed a car that was stopped in the emergency lane. They pulled over, and she and her husband tried to provide help. The woman was standing behind the stalled car. Another car came speeding up from behind, swerved out of its lane, and struck her. Immediately, both legs were amputated. Thanks to some fast first responders, the bleeding was controlled.

When the ambulance brought the woman to the ER, we stabilized her and then transferred her for definitive treatment, prosthesis and extensive rehabilitation. It was wonderful that she had lived, but it seemed ironic that in trying to relieve someone's distress, she had lost both of her legs. I suppose there is a moral buried in that story somewhere.

Another patient comes to mind, and he had chest pain. This gentleman was in his mid-fifties and had experienced left chest pain for about one hour before seeking help. His vital signs were fine and he was alert, however, the EKG (heart tracing) suggested that he was having an acute MI (myocardial infarct or heart attack). We immediately swung into action, establishing IV's, and placing him on the heart monitor. Suddenly, his eyes rolled back and he went into cardio-respiratory arrest in front of us. What a nice coincidence for him, we were all trained for this. We began to assist respirations and perform CPR (cardio-pulmonary resuscitation). He was quickly intubated, given the usual IV meds and responded very well. He quickly became more alert, was extubated, and was admitted.

I saw him walking around a few days later, soon after he was discharged. It is extremely rewarding, both professionally and spiritually, when all of the education actually works and produces a positive outcome.

I remember a nurse that I actively tried to remove from the ER. I have rarely gotten involved with the employment decisions regarding nurses, but she was truly a danger to patients. I was shocked and amazed by her lack of knowledge and poor decision-making skill. This was the scenario. A middle-aged man came to the ER, because he had fallen on a glass table and sustained a large laceration (twenty-five cm) to his left, lateral flank (left side of the abdominal wall). The wound was bleeding profusely and I hurriedly trying to control the hemorrhage. A couple of other staff members were there at the time, including the dangerous nurse I referred to.

At that time, a woman rolled in while CPR was being performed on her. I announced to the nurses, who were helping with the bleeder, that I had to run take care of the Code Blue. They should continue to control the bleeding, I indicated, and I would quickly return. I left and ran the code; the woman died.

I returned to the room with the bleeding man. The nurse who I mistrusted was the only one left in the room. She was documenting his falling blood pressure, but not even trying to control the bleeding with simple pressure. There was now a large pool of blood on the bed next to him, and it had spilled over onto the floor, forming another large pool. I was enraged at the nurse. I screamed that even laypeople knew enough to hold pressure on an actively bleeding laceration. This nurse had worked in the Duke Emergency Department and was always telling war stories of her cases at Duke. I continued my verbal assault, by adding that I had expected much better "from an experienced Duke ER nurse".

I finally gained control of the man's bleeding, and I made certain that the laceration had not penetrated into his abdomen. Unfortunately, now he required some blood transfusions to assist his blood pressure. I repaired his laceration, observed him for a few hours, and then discharged him home.

The next day, I approached the ER nursing supervisor, and explained my position on this particular nurses' behavior. I simply requested that we never be scheduled to work together in the future. I never saw that nurse again.

By now I was getting older, and much more experienced, about thirty years of practice or so. Occasionally it helped. One of the young ER nurses went in to examine a patient who had just arrived from one of the local nursing homes. She took the woman's vital signs, pulse-oximetry and examined the patient. Then she walked out from behind the curtain and pronounced that the patient was stable. I went in, looked at the patient, spent less than a minute, came out and let the nurse know that her patient was dying. She went back in just in time to see the old woman take her last breath. The nurse was shocked, she never seen someone with agonal respirations. The patient had a "do not resuscitate" directive, so it was alright not to proceed with a code.

The nurse was shaken up, and for her next note on the chart she wrote that "COPA was called"(COPA is the agency that harvests corneas and organs if allowed). We all began to laugh and told her that perhaps she would want to "adjust" the chart, since it read that everything was fine and that then COPA was called. Maybe, we suggested, she could add a line after her initial assessment "that the patient had a rapid, downhill course, expired and COPA was called". In reality, while the nurse had been wrong in her initial assessment of the patient, this did not affect or delay any possible treatments for the dying patient. The charting issue was hilarious, however, and the nurse was appropriately chagrined. We teased her mercilessly for hours about that case.

Another ER nurse, very experienced and one of the best I have ever worked with, made an incredibly "not-smart" decision in patient care. An elderly woman presented to the ER, with a large, deep scalp laceration. In general, scalp lacerations bleed heavily, and this one did as well. There was blood everywhere— on the floor, the stretcher and obviously on the patient. I grabbed some hemostats (clamps) and quickly tied off the "bleeders" to control the hemorrhage. It took awhile to repair the scalp laceration, because the woman was demented and uncooperative, but I finally managed to finish the repair. I was standing at the central desk, writing-up her chart, when I heard a "sickening" thud from behind her curtain.

I quickly threw back the curtain to reveal one of our best ER nurses standing over the woman, who had fallen in the floor. The nurse's explanation was that she had directed the patient to stand so she could obtain "orthostatic blood pressures", when the patient collapsed on the floor. I was amazed and did not really understand her actions. In the ER, orthostatic (standing position) blood-pressure changes are often used to determine if a patient's story about blood loss is truly significant. Laypeople often exaggerate the amount of blood actually lost. It is not their fault. They are often excited, and a little bit of blood may appear to them like "a whole lot". We already knew that this woman's blood loss was significant. The blood was everywhere; there was no need to guess.

After a quick exam that did not reveal any additional injuries, we helped the patient back into the bed. I explained to the nurse that we really did not need orthostatic readings this time, since the evidence was overwhelming. The rest of us roared with laughter at her methods.

During another patient encounter, I completely lost my professional attitude. The patient had come to the ER at about four in the morning for chest pain. It had been a very difficult shift and I was extremely tired. I reviewed his chart, which said that his vital signs were normal and he had appeared calm and alert when we first assessed him. As I entered his room, I noticed him lying calmly on the bed with a pack of Camel cigarettes in his shirt pocket. I had already seen on the chart that he had poorly controlled diabetes in his past history. He also had two previous heart attacks, heart bypass surgery, and numerous prior cardiac stents (devices to keep the heart blood vessels open). All of these bits of history are large risk factors for further heart disease.

He began to describe his chest pain and I lost my composure. I became so angry with him that I unleashed a verbal assault. "What do you want the system to do for you, that you are clearly not willing to do for yourself? It is not a matter of *if* you are going to have another heart attack, but only a matter of *when*".

In awhile, I calmed down. I proceeded to take his history and treat him like any other chest pain patient. He never responded to my verbal abuse, and his workup was negative, so he was discharged. I never was clear on exactly what he expected from the medical system.

Many times I have witnessed scenes like the following, and it makes me angry. The paramedics brought in an elderly lady for evaluation of abdominal pain. The paramedics told me about the living conditions at the home, where they found this woman. She was lying on the floor, in her own stool and urine, with a Raid can close to her, to spray any roaches that might approach her. Her daughter was supposed to be caring for her, but she just cashed the monthly social security check and left her mother alone while she went out to "party". Social services had already investigated, but the situation remained. Unfortunately, neglect of the elderly like this was not an isolated incident. It seems impossible to believe that anyone, with a conscience, would treat a family member this way, but they do.

Along this line of thought, another case comes to mind. An elderly gentleman brought his wife to the ED for "leg pain". The patient was an elderly diabetic woman, who had already lost her right leg due to gangrene. She was alert and smiling, but her left leg looked horrible. Below the knee, the bone was exposed with shreds of flesh and muscle clinging to what was left of the leg. It resembled a terrible shark attack. He had been lying next to this woman for weeks and just ignored it. The nurses said the stench was horrible. I was enraged. I asked the husband how he could let this happen to his wife. It obviously had not occurred over just two or three days. He mumbled some excuse. She was admitted and the left leg was amputated. After all these years, human behavior can still baffle me.

I knew it was going to be a rough shift when my first patient was a Code Blue. The paramedics were heroically performing CPR on this man, as they rolled him from the ambulance into the ED. He was an enormous man. We guessed his weight at over five hundred pounds and later found that it was five hundred and sixty pounds. I went to the head, and surprisingly, succeeded in getting him intubated. We started a deep line for IV meds, after a quick, futile search for accessible places to start an IV on his arms. The heart monitor displayed ventricular fibrillation (a very bad heart rhythm with ineffective pumping action). We defibrillated him at the maximum 360 joules, tried various medicines, and repeated defibrillation. I finally stopped the code and pronounced him dead. I really suspect that because of his massive size, the electricity from the paddles could not penetrate through to the heart.

We called for more paramedics to come and help move the body to the morgue. It took six men to move this man. He was only in his early forties.

I went to break the news to his mother. She became hysterical, crying, and screaming. I did not say it out loud, but thought, *You did not really think that your son was healthy, did you?*

I had another difficult case involving a very large man. This patient was very much alive and active— he had overdosed on some kind of stimulant, perhaps methamphetamine, cocaine or both. Eight people, including me, were trying to hold him down as he attempted to hit personnel, bite people, lunge off the stretcher, kick, and in general cause mayhem in the ED. Already in this department there were six or seven other patients, with their own emergencies.

We were trying to administer "medical restraints", a euphemism for sedating medication, but we were not having a lot of luck. The problem here was that if I gave him too much medication, this large patient might not be able to maintain his airway. If I did not give him enough, he could hurt himself or some of the emergency department staff. He weighed more than 500lbs and I was afraid that if I paralyzed him for an intubation, that I might not get the tube in and he would die.

For the first and only time in my career, I requested the on-call anesthesiologist to come help me. He came and inserted the tube with minimal problems; we then used a long-acting paralytic agent to keep the patient secure while whatever drugs he had taken wore off. He did well, but I never found out what he had taken. It must have been a lot, whatever it was.

While we are on the subject, overdose was a common diagnosis, and I ran into another case, later, in another ED. Once again, this patient was a very large male. He had taken some sort of stimulant and fought with everyone that approached him. He was very disruptive, and aggressive. I used "medical restraints" on him also, but despite large doses of sedatives and anti-psychotics, he continued to howl and bark. Finally, he was such a threat to himself and others that I had no choice, but to paralyze and intubate him. It worked. All the drugs wore off, and he left against or medical advice. We never found out what he had taken that produced such bizarre behavior.

In discussing overdose, I should take the opportunity to discuss the state of mental health. I have worked closely with the mental health staff in numerous counties. Almost without exception, I have found them to be extremely dedicated, committed and conscientious people. They, like me, have seen a disturbing trend in the care of the mentally disabled. The funds to help have continued to be cut, while the demands for the services continue to rise. Most of the cases involve attempted suicide, addiction and requests for help, or frank psychoses.

I remember one case vividly. The woman was in her early sixties, and had worked for IBM most of her adult life. She was retired and recently widowed, but she had very attentive and close family members nearby. She had excellent, comprehensive health insurance. She developed an acute psychosis that involved paranoia and visual hallucinations. There are numerous, good anti-psychotic medicines that would help her, and she had attentive family members that would make sure she took her medicine. For a mental health case, her financial and family situation was a gift from God, but no one would accept the patient. Here was a case that the mental health system was made for, and no one would help. The local mental health coordinator finally succeeded in finding a place for her, but it took a long time.

It is not uncommon for these patients to sit in an ED for hours or days, with a local deputy by law, while a bed is found for them. The ED staff's choices are often either releasing the person back to the street or watching them go to jail. The mental health staffs are already stretched very thin, as their work loads increase. It is a problem, and it is getting worse, not better.

A Code Blue involving a child or infant is often a messy, chaotic affair. Pediatric codes are not common, and they are usually the result of some airway problem, followed by cardiac arrest. Everyone gets a excited with these situations. All of the equipment sizes are different, the drug doses are different, and the patients are so small. A man named Broselow invented the Broselow tape to assist in deciding what dose, and what size, but unless the facility is a specialty pediatric emergency department, where these cases are fairly common, these events remain a bit unsettling.

I have been involved in several pediatric codes, over the years, but a few really stand out. One of the local physicians had seen this child in her office and decided to transfer her to Duke for further treatment and evaluation. The problem was acute respiratory distress (difficulty breathing). This doctor was astute enough to doubt whether the child would survive the transfer to Duke, so she sent her to our ED for stabilization. It turned out to be a wise decision, because the child underwent cardio-pulmonary arrest just after arriving in the ER. The mother accompanied the child and was obviously anxious. It seems this child had been born with some sort of congenital abnormality and had required frequent medical interventions in order to survive.

One more time, I shifted into high gear and began trying to help the child. She was about one and a half years old and, of course, cute as a button. I quickly intubated her, and inserted an intra-osseous needle into her tibia (a needle placed in the shinbone)for IV meds and fluids. The intra-osseous needle has been a huge advance forward for ED physicians in trying to care for pediatric patients. The needle is inserted into the bone marrow and almost all IV medicines and fluids may then be delivered. Prior to this, IV access in infants and pediatric patients was very difficult. The child responded well to the code maneuvers. She was then stabilized and transferred to Duke Hospital.

A few weeks later, the mother brought the child to the ER to let me see her and to thank me for helping. That kind of gratitude and recognition is greatly appreciated— and rare— in ED medicine.

Another case did not end as well. This time an obstetrician called a code on a newborn, in the nursery. When I first saw the infant, the OB doctor was already ventilating the intubated infant manually, rhythmically squeezing a bag to send air into the little lungs. I assisted by obtaining the IV access and gave the usual meds, but to no avail. Nothing seemed to help. The OB doctor just kept ventilating the infant. We need to remember that, in the world of Obstetrics, things are usually very happy. The patients all get "better" in 9 months and everyone is usually thrilled with a new baby in the house. I watched this OB doctor continue to ventilate the now dead infant. He was so sad. I finally reached up and told him that he could stop. The infant was dead. He began to softly, quietly, cry. It was heart-wrenching to witness. His patients usually went home and were very happy. He was not used to death.

I saw another case that should be a sharp reminder to all deer hunters, not to go in the woods alone. It was the last day of deer season and this older gentleman left to go to his favorite deer stand. Unfortunately, he went by himself, neglecting to tell anyone where he was going. It was late December, but fortunately it was not too cold. Somehow, he fell out of the deer stand and broke his back in the fall. He lay in the woods and watched the sun come up and go down, while hoping that someone would find him. When he did not come home that evening, his wife began to search for him. She contacted some friends. They started visiting all the places where he usually hunted.

Two days after the hunter fell, they found his car and then found him back in the woods. He was hypothermic (low body temperature) and paralyzed, but alive. The ambulance brought him to the ER, where we warmed him, gave him fluids. We transferred him for more treatment and rehabilitation.

This next case illustrates the value of maintaining an emotionally unattached objectivity, when providing emergency care. The patient was the mother of a coworker at this facility, and I knew this. She presented with signs suggestive of an acute abdomen. The patient was experiencing severe abdominal pain and was screaming and writhing on the bed. With these indications, there are four potential diagnoses that immediately come to the mind of most ER physicians: ruptured abdominal aortic aneurysm, bowel perforation (hole in the bowel wall), small bowel obstruction, and acute mesenteric ischemia (decreased blood flow to the bowel). I was afraid for her because most of those diagnoses do not have a good outcome.

I quickly began to work on her and try to establish the diagnosis. Over the next few hours, I obtained various x-rays, CT scans and lab work trying to pin down a diagnosis, but to no avail. I was astonished! The woman appeared to have an acute abdomen, but all the tests were negative. We finally figured it out. She simply had the Norwalk virus and diarrhea that many people, including me, had suffered through, but she was very frantic and vocal about her discomfort. My impression of her had been distorted because of the connection that I had with her daughter. The on-call physician admitted her for IV fluids and observation. She did well and was discharged home the next day.

Eventually, at this small-town emergency room, I treated my last patients, and retired. While I thought I was done with my patients, it turned out that a patient's relatives were not yet done with me. Shortly after I retired from active practice, I received notice of my third—and hopefully last—lawsuit. This case made me angry.

It involved a woman in her mid-thirties who had been seen by me for cough and cold symptoms. Her work-up, including blood work and chest x-ray, had all been negative. Her pulse oximetry value (blood oxygen level) was normal at 98%. My patient was alert, talking to all the staff, and specifically denied having any chest pain three different times. Her vital signs were all normal, except for a slightly elevated temperature of 99. She had no past medical history and her only meds were some birth control pills.

Two weeks after I saw her, she had a large pulmonary embolus (blood clot to the lungs) and died. In the two-week interval, she had seen another doctor, who also found nothing of concern.

The deceased woman's survivors sued me, along with several others, for malpractice. At the advice of my attorney, we settled out of court. He explained to me that the company had already calculated the break-even amount for a settlement, considering retainer fees and court costs.

The hardest part was yet to come. I was told that the young woman's parents would get the money. It seems that they had abandoned the girl, when she was two, and she had been raised by her aunts. The parents did not live together, and only occasionally saw their daughter. I was truly sorry that the girl had died, but I was not sure that it was my fault, and now the system was going to make her absent surviving parents rich. Some system!

CHAPTER 8

Final Thoughts

WHAT DID I LEARN AFTER ALL those years in the ER? It is a time-worn cliché, and a universal truth, that needs to be relearned frequently. *Life truly is precious, and so very brief.* The Roman's had a phrase –carpe diem- or "seize the day". It is still applicable today. It is so easy to become distracted by the mundane problems of everyday life. Life is hard. That is just the way it is. But with touch, understanding and compassion, we all have the capacity to make this journey of life so much better for each other. This is what I learned in the ER. Something that all of us already know.

I have one last story to share that dramatically demonstrates just how brief and precious life truly is. I was talking to a paramedic friend of mine years ago. I was about 35 years old and so was he. We were both young, full of life and promise. He loved to ride his motorcycle. We finished talking and he left to go home. I saw him again in the ER, about an hour later. He was now a trauma victim from a wreck. He was dead. He had no face. He was a wonderful person.

I have tried to apply these lessons in my own life. I am currently writing in the jungles of Costa Rica, where I am surrounded by tropical flowers, toucans, hummingbirds, Howler monkeys, and overlooking the Pacific Ocean. I have been fortunate enough to have hiked the Canadian Rockies, with their alpine meadows and snow-capped mountains. I have seen the Aurora Borealis in Alaska, and been scuba diving all over the Caribbean and South Pacific. I have been skiing in the Colorado Rockies, and biked along the Blue Ridge Parkway. These are things that bring me great pleasure, and even though I am not wealthy, I did not wait to experience them.

There is a growing problem with the medical system as it exists today. The discovery of new technologies has been spectacular. But combined with the increased beaurocratic demands, it comes at a cost. Doctors don't have the time to listen to patients and touch them. I have experienced this myself as a patient and I hear it often in conversations with people. Touch and listening are necessary for patients to feel better, when they are sick or dying. This is probably the art of medicine.

I have already revealed my feelings about the malpractice tort system as it exists today. It has its place, but it is flawed. Undoubtedly, through litigation, many incompetent physicians have been revealed and removed from practice. When I hear a story about the wrong leg being amputated or surgical instruments being left in someone's body, I can not help but wince. These events are wrong and some sort of punishment is completely appropriate.

However, when a potential malpractice case comes to be regarded as a possible "lottery win", I think the pendulum has swung too far to one side. When every new patient encounter is viewed as a potential litigation case, the focus is less on the illness and more on avoiding the lawyers. This is a regrettable situation for our society. The legal profession, acting with the labor unions, has achieved wondrous goals for the working man's rights in this country. Lawyers have also achieved wondrous goals for patient's rights, but perhaps it is time to review our current position.

I have talked a lot about death, in these chapters. It is a subject that is often neglected, for obvious reasons. No one enjoys discussing death, but it is a conversation that many people need to hear. Death is inevitable. There is a phenomenon known as "*death with dignity*" and, in my opinion, it is time to bring it back. Society's expectations of the medical system have greatly exceeded its ability to deliver. Medicine has come a long way, but the goal of achieving increased longevity and providing quality of life, still eludes medicine. I remember viewing my first CT scan, and marveling at the images. I have also witnessed great progress in the treatments of diabetes, cardiovascular diseases and hypertension to name a few, but the nursing homes are full of patients who are still alive, but no longer have any quality of life left.

I have spent my career trying to cheat or delay death. Many times, I have received an elderly patient, from some nursing home, who has no quality of life left. They often have contracted limbs, dementia, and can't walk or talk.

They have a feeding tube placed for sustenance, a catheter in their bladder to void, and have existed in this condition for years. Their family members have not visited them in months, and the patient would not know it if they did come. However, if the patient should experience cardiac arrest (heart stops), the family will communicate, by phone, that *"you should do everything"*. I often think, *do you really want us to do all the painful procedures to this person, so that, if they live, they can return to the nursing home.* What an enormous waste of money and resources.

I, personally, do not want to be the one making the decisions, but we as a society need to do just that. I am not certain of the specific numbers, but I have often read that about 80% of the health-care dollars that exist are spent during the last two years of life. Personally, I would rather see the money spent on pediatrics, to extend a child's life or possibly cure him or her. If there were unlimited health-care dollars, then the decision would be moot, but the health-care dollars are limited, and we as a society are going to have to make choices. This is not about *"death panels"*, but rather the intelligent allocation of a very finite resource.

I have quit the practice of medicine now and returned to my beloved mountains. Now, I am living out the *"Green Acres"* (an old TV sitcom about leaving the big city and trying to live on a farm) lifestyle and enjoying it immensely. The practice of Medicine has changed drastically over the last decade; I have failed to change with it. In my opinion, it has evolved into just another business, with the emphasis on profit, not quality.

I grew tired of the constant e-mails from "corporate" that *I did not make them enough money* during the preceding month. They insisted that I had not practiced "bad" medicine, but that I did not make them enough money. The not-so-veiled suggestion was that I should try ordering more unnecessary laboratory work or admitting more patients without medical justification, since that is where the money is located. I even had one conversation, in which I was told that "*you no longer see patients, Dr. Bentley— you see customers*".

I know that I am a "dinosaur", but I still believe in the existence of *patients*, so I quit. These are just my opinions, but I don't think that medicine can be run like just any other business. Now, when I hear the siren scream, I think to myself "*they are playing my song, but they are not coming to me anymore*". I suppose that I will miss the steady stream of human pathology, and the "chorus" of croup coughs in children; but probably not much.

I have spent the past few pages trying to convey the feelings and passion that occur in the practice of emergency medicine in this country. These are only my experiences and my perspective. Many of the stories from one ER to the next are similar, but each physician experiences these circumstances in his or her own way.

It may be said that it is better to read about what happens in an ER, than to have to visit one with an emergency. I hope these stories have revealed the very real world of emergency medicine.